Two Minu chological

Two Minute Talks to Improve Psychological and Behavioral Health

JOHN F. CLABBY

PhD

Clinical Associate Professor of Family Medicine and Psychiatry
Robert Wood Johnson Medical School (RWJMS)
University of Medicine and Dentistry of New Jersey (UMDNJ)
Behavioral Scientist
Family Medicine Residency and Geriatric Fellowship Programs
CentraState Medical Center
Freehold, NJ

Foreword by

KENNETH W. FAISTL

MD, FAAFP

Associate Professor of Family Medicine
Robert Wood Johnson Medical School (RWJMS)
University of Medicine and Dentistry of New Jersey (UMDNJ)
Director, Family Medicine Residency Program
CentraState Medical Center
Freehold, NJ

Radcliffe Publishing
London • New York

Radcliffe Publishing Ltd
33–41 Dallington Street
London
EC1V 0BB
United Kingdom

www.radcliffepublishing.com
Electronic catalogue and worldwide online ordering facility.

British Library Cataloguing in Publication Data
A catalogue record for this book is available from the British Library.

ISBN-13: 978 184619 369 9

The paper used for the text pages of this book
is FSC® certified. FSC (The Forest Stewardship
Council®) is an international network to promote
responsible management of the world's forests.

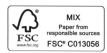

Typeset by Pindar NZ, Auckland, New Zealand
Printed and bound by TJI Digital, Padstow, Cornwall, UK

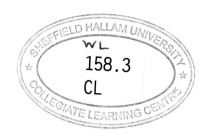

Contents

Foreword

For the better part of 35 years, I have practiced Family Medicine in a community hospital, providing care to varying populations in traditional clinical practice, in a correctional facility, youth home, substance abuse residential treatment and, most recently, as an educator of Family Physicians. The challenges have been to say the least, interesting; trying to bridge my own life experiences and those of others under my care has been an area where little of my formal education has helped. Relying on small snippets of other's tales of success is frankly the only guidance and direction that was available to me.

Dr. Clabby in his book *Two Minute Talks to Improve Psychological and Behavioral Health* develops plans demonstrating to individuals some techniques and examples that could be incorporated into their personal approach, allowing them to close the distance between patients and providers. Organized into chapters that reference what I have seen as repetitive, often deteriorating, personal behavior patterns in patients, Dr. Clabby provides a strategy for recognition and intervention that validates the fact that learning from other's experience can be successful in avoiding anxiety turning into panic or loss of control evolving into depression. Failure to recognize a problem results in a lost opportunity to treat, with the result often a worse potential outcome. Engaging patients reduces barriers to treatment.

I have been fortunate to watch the techniques discussed actually practiced, while Dr. Clabby treats, teaches and shares his experience with student physicians, nurses, psychologists and social workers. I have personally witnessed his care of vulnerable populations, using the short, evidence-based skills outlined. This book is a culmination of techniques that have extended capabilities to many students while they learn to "close the distance" between patient and provider, creating a positive treatment environment. This illustration will make you understand that turning an empathetic professional into a skilled clinician is possible. It will "reveal" to you talents and results you did not believe possible.

It will re-energize your approach to care, and make it fun to talk with and get to know your patients.

Kenneth W. Faistl MD, FAAFP
Associate Professor of Family Medicine
Robert Wood Johnson Medical School
Director, Family Medicine Residency Program
CentraState Medical Center
Freehold, NJ
January 2011

Preface

Many healthcare professionals avoid asking their patients about their psycho-social lives. Beyond recommending medication consultations, it is difficult to know what else to do with the stories they hear. There are also concerns about opening a Pandora's Box of unmanageable conversations that will be time inefficient. This needs to change. Undiagnosed, under-treated emotional upset causes expensive debilitating injury to the body as well as to the mind. It just does not have to be this way. Much can be competently addressed even with two minute talks.

One of the challenges in writing this narrative is the dual way in which our culture regards the way to provide psychological and behavioral healthcare. At one extreme it is believed that almost anyone who has good interpersonal skills, and who is kind and empathic, is ready to provide the kind of healing that is required in this work. At the other extreme it is held that this is a complex field which is so ripe for practitioner error that only the most highly trained professional should undertake this. This book attempts to split this difference by avoiding a denseness or hidden language that would make it impenetrable to those who are not mental health insiders, or that would require years of training to implement. Make no mistake about it, we need mental health insiders. As a psychologist who has been working in private clinical practice for over 30 years, I am one of them. The matters discussed in this book are quite serious, and I do not minimize that. For example, the narrative frequently refers to the importance of making a referral to a physician to rule out physical illness or to consider medication. However, the truth is that because of personal preferences or access issues, many people tell their troubles to those whose primary responsibility is in areas other than psychological and behavioral health. They may bring personal concerns to a physician after discussing diabetes management, to a dental professional after undergoing a procedure, to a co-worker after a department meeting, or to a friend while picking up a child from school. These are not mental health insiders. They save lives by adjusting diabetes medications, treating painful dental cavities, managing complex offices, or being friends who care. A variation on the ancient proverb captures it well – when the troubled person is ready, the advisor will appear. The world cannot afford to disenfranchise the many adults who, with additional information, can begin to relieve psychological and behavioral suffering with two minute talks.

I have seen such brief encounters happen many times in my work training family physicians. I have witnessed doctors save a marriage (by recommending that the couple keep calm for the first 15 minutes after saying hello, because this sets a lasting tone), reduce depression (by moving someone from misery talk to positive talk), and activate healthy eating (by asking what would be fun to do when the weight has been lost). These changes were facilitated by brief therapeutic observations, bits of advice, and activating questions that are all examples of many evidence-based interventions described in this book.

There are important books that provide significant detail regarding the research underpinnings that support specific advising and counseling approaches. That is not the focus of this book. This text is written for those who have little time and possibly little interest in extensive primary source study and reading. There are important books that focus a full effort on a painful emotion such as depression or panic. Frankly, however, many troubled people do not directly present with such complaints. Instead, they speak about marital stress, anxiety about making an oral presentation, dealing with a mean-spirited co-worker, poor nutritional habits, handling uncooperative children or early adolescents, and domestic violence. They want practical guidance about those content areas as well. So this book addresses not only the traditional emotional topics but also the real-life, everyday problems that underlie those toxic feelings, yet which are so rarely addressed.

I have made an effort to write in a style that is inviting, not intimidating. I have strived to offer recommendations that are clear and accessible, and to avoid the vague, dense, and unrealistic recommendations that marginalize mental health insiders and caricature us as eccentric and out of touch. For those readers who want to learn more, many references are made to helpful sources and resources.

The topics selected for this book are based upon the problems that commonly present to family physicians, problems that commonly present to me in my clinical practice, and often draw upon the formal lectures and grand rounds that I have provided to family medicine residents.

The book is organized around the following six sections. Section 1 is on 'Practical strategies from powerful psychotherapies.' Writing this section was a significant challenge to the goal of making the book inviting and practical. Respectfully summarizing the key tenets of several psychotherapeutic schools was a formidable challenge. However, I feel good about how it turned out and about the fact that I included this material at the very beginning. While it is important to grow competency in certain problem content areas, such as alcohol use, it is also important to be grounded in how to communicate in ways that facilitate therapeutic change. A reader who wants to help clients to stop bullying themselves by their negative self-talk can focus on cognitive therapy. The reader who is interested in helping clients to learn to solve their own problems can concentrate on social problem solving. The solution-focused advising section shows how to move clients from misery talk to positive talk. Those readers who want to help clients to change to healthy habits such as nicotine abstinence can spend time on motivational advising.

Section 2 is titled straightforwardly, 'Eating, sleeping, smoking, and drinking.' These are four of the most common problems that concern physical and behavioral health providers. The recommendations that are made take the advisor well beyond the often used and yet often unsuccessful approach of providing mini-lectures to clients about knowledge that they already have. The narrative makes an effort to help clients to recognize and accept that they are quite able to make simple and effective changes.

Section 3 is concerned with 'Managing stress, panic, and depression.' It starts with an epidemiological look at the prevalence of stress, and then teaches a simple intervention of IBM – imagery, breathing, and muscle relaxation. Gaining control over panic comes next, and is followed by screening for unipolar depression, and how to manage this problem, as well as how not to miss bipolar depression.

Section 4 is on 'Marriages, relationships, children, and teens.' The number one reason why adults give up their evenings at home and seek the help of mental health professionals is because they are concerned about their troubled marriages and relationships, and because they are struggling with their children and teenagers. Practical ways to understand such relationships as well as practical strategies are provided.

Section 5, on 'Bad news, violence, and grieving', discusses how to humanely deliver disappointing news, ranging from a job loss to a divorce to a death in the family. This is followed by advice regarding violence against women, as well as a very brief observation on identifying young people who are at risk for violence. The section closes with a presentation on dispelling the myths about grieving, and presents guidance on healthy grieving.

Section 6, 'Thriving at work', focuses on maintaining a positive attitude at work. This is a crucial element which, if not attended to, creates major emotional problems. The emphasis here is on handling the pressures of taking on leadership and supervisory responsibilities, learning how to provide feedback effectively, handling difficult and critical co-workers, and speaking up effectively in groups.

John F. Clabby
January 2011

About the author

John F. Clabby, PhD is a Clinical Associate Professor of Family Medicine and Community Health and Psychiatry at the University of Medicine and Dentistry of New Jersey (UMDNJ) – Robert Wood Johnson Medical School (RWJMS), CentraState Family Medicine Residency and Geriatric Fellowship Programs in Freehold, New Jersey. He also holds a joint appointment with the Rutgers University Graduate School of Applied Professional Psychology. Dr. Clabby is a NJ Licensed Psychologist. Prior to joining the Family Medicine faculty at RWJMS, he was Chief Psychologist for the University of Medicine and Dentistry of New Jersey–University Behavioral Healthcare, where he was the Director of the Social Decision-Making/Social Problem Solving Program.

Dr. Clabby has co-authored three books with Dr. Maurice Elias, authored many articles and chapters, and given numerous lectures on practical strategies to promote mental health. Over the years, periodicals such as *US News and World Report*, the *New York Times*, and the *Journal of the American Medical Association* have written about his work. Dr. Clabby has won several national awards including the National Mental Health Association's Lela Rowland Prevention Award, the American Psychological Association's National Psychological Consultants to Management Award, and the National Psychology Award for Excellence in the Media, Book Category (Honorable Mention). He has twice been nominated for the Outstanding Seminar Award at the Society of Teachers of Family Medicine NE Annual Conference. A much sought-after speaker, Dr. Clabby maintains a private clinical psychotherapy practice in the Monmouth County, New Jersey area near the ocean beaches where he grew up, and where he and his wife raised their four children.

Acknowledgments

I am fortunate to be on the faculty of the CentraState Family Medicine Residency and Geriatric Fellowship Programs – University of Medicine and Dentistry of New Jersey (UMDNJ) – Robert Wood Johnson Medical School (RWJMS) in Freehold, New Jersey. The following colleagues make coming to work each morning a pleasure. They teach me what I need to know and provide unquestioned support. They are: Kenneth W. Faistl, MD, FAAFP, a visionary leader who makes great ideas a reality, and Maria Ciminelli, MD, who brilliantly champions the biopsychosocial model of care at the highest level. When the ideas presented in this book seem sensible and practical, it is because of what I have learned from my extraordinary colleagues at CentraState: Lisa Mellor, MD; Joshua Raymond, MD, MPH, CMD; Robert Chen, MD, MBA; Alicia R. Dermer, MD, FABM, IBCLC; Bennett S. Shenker, MD, MSPH; Geronima Alday, MD; Steve Weintraub, DO; Karen W. Foster, RN, MSA; Liz Donahue, RN, BSN; Lynn Schwenzer, MHSA; Kelly Dallavalle, BS; Jodi Franklin, BA; Paula Doll, CSW; Nannette Asuncion, RN, APN; Barbara Giannone, BS, RD (who advised me about healthy eating); Laurie Huryk, RN, BSN; Maryellen Dykeman, RN, MSN, TDTS (who advised me about smoking cessation); Taru Sinha, MD; Adity Bhattacharyya, MD, FAAFP; Sonia Garcia Laumbach, MD; the Family Medicine Center's outstanding nursing staff, reception staff, and our fantastic and dedicated family medicine resident physicians.

I extend my heartfelt appreciation to John T. Gribbin, President and CEO of the CentraState Healthcare System; Dan Messina, PhD, FACHE, LNHA, Senior Vice President and Chief Operating Officer; Ben Weinstein, MD, PhD, Senior Vice President and Chief Medical Officer; the Board of Trustees and the dedicated administrative and clinical staff of our hospital system. I would especially like to thank Robin Siegel, MLS, AHIP, CentraState's Medical Librarian, for her conscientious, responsive professionalism in locating references. I also thank Gillian Nineham, Editorial Director at Radcliffe Publishing, who first saw the promise of this book at a Society of Teachers of Family Medicine NE Conference in Baltimore, as well as the other professionals at Radcliffe Publishing including Michael Hawkes, Jamie Etherington, Jessica Morofke, and Martin Hill who all skilfully shepherded this book through the process. I also thank my colleagues at RWJMS, in particular our Department Chair, Alfred Tallia, MD, MPH, who encourages our efforts at scholarship. In addition I thank David Swee, MD, who first brought me onto faculty at RWJMS, and honored me with the opportunity to learn from Marian Stuart, PhD. I also thank the Behavioral Scientists Group of the RWJMS Network of Family Medicine Residencies, as well as my fellow faculty members at UMDNJ–RWJMS and University Behavioral Healthcare, who taught me so much from the very beginning. I benefit from the loyal and confident support provided by Lauren, Jimmy, Jackson, Jack, Katie, Nora, Sheila, David, Patrick, Kristine, my parents John Francis Clabby and Virginia Dolan Clabby, my extended family of brothers, and brothers-in-law, sisters and sisters-in-law, nieces, nephews, and friends, particularly Bob Hochreiter. I especially acknowledge Lauren Clabby Moore, whose skillful editing brought a directness and clarity to this narrative. Most importantly, I thank Wendy Melone Clabby for her generous sacrifices to support this evening, vacation day, and weekend writing project, her scholarly and technical contributions, and for inspiring me with her compassion for the afflicted.

For Wendy Melone Clabby

Practical strategies from powerful psychotherapies

CLIENT STRENGTHS, ADVISOR–CLIENT RAPPORT, AND POSITIVE EXPECTATIONS

People want to talk to someone who can help them with their behavioral and psychological troubles. The person who gives the help is in some circles called the doctor, the psychologist, the counselor, the mentor, or the coach, and in this book is referred to as the advisor. The person receiving the help could be called the patient, the customer, or the consumer, and in this book is called the client.

In a poll conducted by *Newsweek*, nearly 20% of adults in the U.S. reported that they had had some form of psychotherapy or counseling, and 4% were currently in therapy.[1] A study of 14,000 households found that 3.2% of American adults in 1987 and 3.6% in 1997 sought psychotherapy annually.[2]

Those fortunate ones are able to obtain formal psychotherapy. Yet today, as well as throughout the ancient history of men and women, and certainly well before the development of the modern era of trained psychotherapists, there has been a rich tradition of a hidden service of psychotherapy and counseling. These are the brief, two minute talks that clients continue to have with people who are often wise elders, who serve as advisors. These talks, which often last around two minutes, have stood the test of time.

What comes from the current study of psychotherapy for behavioral and psychological health that can make such two minute talks even more effective? The scientific literature on the effectiveness of psychotherapy provides some leads. There is no longer any equivocation. The truth is that psychotherapy and counseling work. However, what makes experiences like psychotherapy work has less to do with unique contributions provided by different psychotherapeutic theories, and more to do with factors that are common to all psychotherapies.[3] Michael Lambert[4] cites four characteristics of all effective psychotherapies and ranks them in order of influence. These are the quality of the personal and environmental strengths that the client already has, the quality of the client–advisor relationship, the power of the placebo effect in building hope and positive expectancies, and finally the technique that the advisor uses.

The quality of the client's personal and environmental strengths counts for 40% of the reason why clients get better after therapeutic talks. These strengths include the client's determination to get better, their personal commitment to the advising experience, their being aware of having successfully resolved such problems before, and/or their having a meaningful spiritual life. Advisors should notice and reinforce such qualities by complimenting clients on having the maturity and courage to ask for advice in the first place. The advisor can reinforce the client's determination by acknowledging the client's energy that is already being put into figuring things out. The advisor can express admiration for the client's commitment to lessening the emotional pain by reaching out. Other environmental factors that influence whether a client makes progress in psychotherapy or advising include having a job that is satisfying, maintaining a connection with an understanding best friend, or reacting positively to chance events such as a favorite team winning a football game. An advisor can notice these factors and comment that such ingredients are significant, hopeful, positive markers.

The healing nature of the client–advisor relationship has repeatedly and in different settings been reported to be the most important component of care.[5] Some researchers argue that the relationship is therapy in its own right, rather than just a communication vehicle through which the real formal therapy works.[6] The quality of the connection between the client and the advisor accounts for about 30% of the reason why clients benefit from one-to-one therapeutic talks. Cultivating and projecting a sense of caring, empathy, warmth, and acceptance is essential to facilitating emotional and behavioral change in a client. This is one of the factors over which advisors have some control, and significant attention needs to be given to learning how to make authentic connections and build rapport.

The power of the placebo effect in building the client's hopes and positive expectancies about the advisor's skills accounts for approximately 15% of the reason why clients benefit from advising. Hope is about a client's expectation that talking with the advisor will lead to success in attaining a personally meaningful and realistic goal (e.g. being happier in a marriage). A client's hope is also based on the client believing that it is possible to achieve the goal, and it is fueled by such advisor and client attributes as energy, resilience and courage, and the availability of important external resources (e.g. having insurance to cover the costs of marital therapy if it is needed). Hope has four components that the advisor can cultivate:

1 emotions, such as encouraging client trust and confidence in the advisor, making the conversation a positive one because it also includes some small talk and even some appropriate humor
2 intellect, such as the advisor encouraging the client to reflect upon past experiences, to set goals, to plan, and to assess the likelihood of success
3 behaviors, such as the advisor encouraging the client's motivation to act positively
4 environmental attributes, such as the resourcefulness of the advisor in locating resources such as low-cost marital therapy if there is no insurance coverage, or connecting the client with a support group.[7]

Advisors will also build hope and positive expectations by growing their expertise about the common life and psychological challenges which they can share with clients. People hold advisors in high regard. They will approach an advisor because of his or her social and occupational status. People trust an advisor because of the advisor's education, training, and professional experience.[8] Projecting confidence without arrogance is a key component to effective advising.

With regard to the technique or the model of treatment that the advisor uses, both the quality of the procedure used and how well the advisor explains the rationale account for 15% of the client's improvement.

In summary, the research recommends that advisors comment on the client's maturity in asking for help, cultivate the connection and rapport, raise the client's expectations that the advice will help, and raise the quality of the advice by maintaining a continuing education effort to learn about problem-specific content areas. Combining these four elements makes the advisor a powerful agent of positive change.

HEARING THE FULL STORY

Since 30% of the success of therapeutic conversations is explained by the relationship and rapport between advisor and client, how can an advisor establish a positive relationship? Many advisors can recall going to someone for help themselves, perhaps even a healthcare professional, and being disappointed by the lack of connection. Despite an advisor's considerable interpersonal and professional skills, sincere listening cannot be faked. Qualities such as humility, sincerity, hopefulness, likeability, and even a healthy sense of humor can be a base for rapport. But what are the technical tasks that can support the work of the advisor? These include eliciting the client's perspective, helping the client to feel understood, explaining what may be happening and what the options might be, handling differences of opinion with grace and care, coming to an optimistic agreement about options that will really help, and using words that are practical and accessible.[9] Excellent rapport starts with a commitment to be fully available to help this client during the conversation.

Active listening starts with authentic belief that the client has an important story to tell. The client has been working up the confidence to talk for some time. At the beginning of the conversation, the advisor must remain calm and let the story come to them. Stuart and Lieberman[10] advise healthcare providers that the first few minutes belong to the patient. The job of the advisor is to create a safe environment and then get out of the way so that the client can tell the story. The wise advisor holds back on questions, suggestions, interpretations, and interventions until the story is completed. Otherwise the client will be preoccupied with wondering whether there will be a chance to tell the tale, and therefore cannot concentrate on any advice, however brilliant, that they are given. Once the client has had a few minutes to tell the story, the advisor may be tempted to ask a series of closed questions: Who were you with? When did this actually happen? What time was it? The effort to get the facts is well intended, but for the client it can be an uncomfortable interrogation, and they may shut down.

At the beginning of the conversation in particular, the advisor should avoid asking closed questions. These are questions that ask for a single word or brief response. For example, the answer to the question "Are you still with Adam?" might just be a "Yes." A skilled advisor uses invitational, open-ended statements, such as "Tell me what's been happening with you and Adam", "Describe the situation", or "Talk to me", along with open-ended questions such as "What happened?" or "What was going on?" Mixing such invitational, open-ended statements with invitational, open-ended questions provides a superior experience. Clients often respond to open-ended statements and questions with many of the details that the advisor would ask for in a closed question anyway. The advisor does not have to work quite so hard, and the client is more actively engaged. Closed questions may be best used as follow-up to obtain additional detail later in the conversation, after the client has had the chance to tell the full story. In addition, clients who feel that they have told their story are also more receptive to the advisor's suggestions when they come up later.

Early on in the conversation, advisors should also avoid asking the "Why?" and "How come?" questions. These can be perceived as evaluative, challenging and invasive. A better way of obtaining more information is to use the two inquiry rule. For example, a client may say "My husband is not interested in my work life." Rather than asking the challenging question "Why do you think that?", the advisor might say "Tell me more about that." This is more inviting in tone and gets the client to dig a little more fully, and possibly more honestly express what is really going on.

AUTHENTIC AND ACTIVE LISTENING

Advisors can enhance rapport by combining a genuine commitment to listen with an interpersonal comportment that reflects this. To this end, advisors should consider the domains of APLUS.[11] This refers to:

➤ Active listening, where the advisor energetically paraphrases the client's thoughts and feelings, demonstrating that listening and not merely hearing is going on

➤ Posture, which is such that the advisor is also seated, relaxed, directly facing the client, perhaps leaning in, and the muscular comportment is steady and calm

➤ Language used, which is an everyday language, free of jargon, and in a quantity that allows for the majority of the words in the dialogue balloon to belong to the client

➤ Use of our eyes, which is such that the advisor, to the extent that is culturally appropriate, listens with their eyes, and looks directly, respectfully, and mutually comfortably at the client

➤ Sound of the voice, where the voice tone is used like a musical instrument to convey a full range from a compassionate-sounding to a business-like tone, based on the current need.

Keeping APLUS in mind, the advisor can self-monitor the key social comportment skills that broadcast sincerity.

The quality of the advisor's listening skills directly builds rapport which facilitates positive, healthy change for the client. The *neurolinguistic programming (NLP)* concept of mirroring helps in this regard. John Grinder and Richard Bandler studied the posture, language, use of eyes, and tone of voice utilised by such expert therapists as Milton Erickson (a hypnotherapist and psychiatrist), Fritz Perls (a psychotherapist), Virginia Satir (a family therapist), and Gregory Bateson (an anthropologist and social psychologist).[12] For example, in their research Grinder and Bandler observed that Ms. Satir matched her choice of verbs, adverbs, and adjectives to those of her patients. Further research revealed that such verbal mirroring was common to the language artistry used by all four of these master psychotherapists.

An advisor can practice mirroring in the following way. In the Speech domain, an inexperienced advisor might interrupt with comments like "OK", "I see", "Uh huh", etc. Unfortunately, those expressions can be interpreted as too casual, appear disingenuous and cost the advisor and client a valuable opportunity to build rapport. Some degree of quietness on the part of the advisor can actually be soothing. In addition, an appropriate use of eye contact, as determined by the other person's culture, also demonstrates the advisor's genuine interest in the patient's unique story.

Paraphrasing and verbal mirroring are among the tools that NLP offers. When advisors paraphrase, they edit and summarize the client's words. This can be a very useful alternative to the "OK", "I see", "Uh huh" approach. At the same time, repeating too many of the client's words or paraphrasing too often interrupts the story too much and also risks distortion. Verbal mirroring includes approximating the sound of the client's voice (e.g. soft or business-like, etc.), repeating the client's last few words or word, and occasionally using a slight questioning inflection. This verbal mirroring avoids distorting the client's words, and often encourages them to say more.

The following is an example of how verbal mirroring builds rapport. Here the advisor shows little energy and simply nods his/her head or states "OK."

Advisor:	Do you have trouble sleeping?
Client:	No, I'm OK with that.
Advisor:	OK (and/or head nod). Have you lost interest in doing things that give you pleasure?
Client:	No.
Advisor:	OK (and/or head nod). Do you feel guilty about anything?
Client:	Not really.
Advisor:	OK (and/or head nod). How is your energy?
Client:	Low.
Advisor:	OK (and/or head nod). Have you ever thought of harming yourself or committing suicide?
Client:	Never.
Advisor:	OK. (and/or head nod). Are you able to concentrate and focus?

The client redundantly sees the same head nod and series of "OK's" to questions about sleep, pleasurable activities, guilt, energy, and self-destructive and suicidal thoughts. To the client, the advisor appears to be more interested in going through a standard list of questions than in understanding the client's concerns, and even seems bored.

Here is an example of the same advisor using verbal mirroring with a questioning inflection of the voice tone. This talk may go as follows.

Advisor:	Do you have trouble sleeping?
Client:	No, I'm OK with that.
Advisor:	You're OK with that. (Pause) Have you lost interest in doing things that give you pleasure?
Client:	No.
Advisor:	No? (Pause) Do you feel guilty about anything?
Client:	No. Not really.
Advisor:	Not really. (Pause) Have you ever thought of harming yourself or committing suicide?
Client:	Never.
Advisor:	Never? (Pauses)
Client:	Well I used to say I'd never try and harm myself, but lately I'm not so sure.

When the advisor repeats the single word "Never" and then pauses, it reminds the client of the emotion underlying the choice of the word "Never." This gives the client the chance to explain whether the word "Never" was significant. When the client elaborates, the advisor really hears what is going on, and rapport is deepened.

Rapport is also enhanced with physical mirroring. As mentioned earlier, Milton Erickson, MD, was a renowned psychiatrist and master hynotherapist. As a polio patient, he was significantly restricted in his physical movements. Yet he became an absolute and legendary master of building rapport by subtly mirroring his client's posture. In mirroring his clients, Dr. Erickson would not directly imitate the client. He would, for example, simply tilt his head at an angle similar to the angle of his client, and respond with subtle physical movements similar to those being used at that moment by his client. It is important to understand the difference between imitating and mirroring. Imitating is obvious and may actually lessen rapport. If a client crosses their left leg over their right leg, an imitator would do the same by crossing the left leg over the right. However, an advisor using mirroring would do the opposite, by crossing the right leg over the left, as if the client were looking in the mirror. The advisor's mirroring actions should lag behind the client's by several seconds to a minute or so.

MANAGING TIME

Managing time within these talks is necessary because if the conversation continues for too long, the advisor will be less likely to want to advise this client or others in the future. This would be a loss for the many clients who could be helped.

The sooner an advisor generates good rapport with a client, the sooner a reservoir of good will is established with that client. The advisor can draw on this reservoir later to respectfully interrupt and redirect the client if there is a need to economize time. Paradoxically, to be time-efficient, the advisor needs to slow down and establish rapport by beginning with some brief socialization. The advisor should offer a social handshake such as a warm greeting (e.g. "It's great to see you again"). If the conversation is beginning later than planned, the advisor can cultivate rapport by politely acknowledging this (e.g. "Thanks for waiting for my call" or "I appreciate your patience"). And the advisor should demonstrate an attentive posture and culturally appropriate eye contact, ensure the client's physical comfort with regard to sitting or standing, and assure them of privacy during the talk.

The advisor should next ascertain the client's agenda for the talk. As reported in the medical literature, "Soliciting the patient's agenda takes little time and can improve interview efficiency and yield increased data."[13] Doctors who let their patients tell their story often have briefer interviews. One family physician reports that "Studies have shown that the patient normally speaks for 18 seconds before the doctor interrupts. But if the doctor lets them speak for three to four minutes, they tell you 90% of what's wrong with them."[14]

Identifying and honoring what the client wants to discuss has significant consequences for time management: "Physicians often redirect patients' initial descriptions of their concerns. Once re-directed, the descriptions are rarely completed. What are the consequences? Late-rising concerns and missed opportunities to gather potentially important patient data."[15]

The advisor needs to make an effort to understand what the client's real issue is, and to confirm this understanding with the client. After the client has taken a minute or so to share the story, the advisor can ask such questions as:

> "Am I right that your number one issue is . . .?"
> "Of all the things you mentioned, what is your top concern?"
> "If we could discuss only one of your issues today, which one would it be?"
> "Wow, you are certainly dealing with a lot of issues. That must be difficult. Let's start with the two most important things, and then we'll see if we have enough time for the rest."
> "How can I best help you today?"

Despite the advisor's best efforts to establish maximum rapport, some clients may still avoid speaking about what is really on their mind. They may be anxious about whether they can trust themselves and/or the advisor to handle the real concern. The client may be testing the advisor's capacity to handle the matter with care and regard. This happens to even the most seasoned and trusted psychotherapists. A sign that this could be happening is when the emotion that the client expresses does not match the story that the advisor is hearing. Or the story may be particularly hard to follow or understand, as if important details are not being mentioned. Advisors should trust their instincts about this and gently ask some slightly more invasive questions, such as:

> "Tell me again what led you to give me a call?"
> "Can you run it by me again, the reasons you wanted us to talk?"
> "We will both benefit from this . . . what is your honest opinion about what is going on?"
> "What is your main concern about what you have started telling me?"
> "Are others who are close to you worried about something in particular?"
> "What about all this particularly concerns you?"
> "What do you think might happen if things don't change?"
> "I'll certainly try and give you some good advice if I can, but first, what do you think ought to happen?"

Sometimes the advisor may discover that the problem at hand is too complex for this one particular talk. In this case, the main goal would be to identify the problem and schedule another time to talk. Once the advisor understands the size and scope of the main concern, time can be rationed appropriately. The advisor can use comments such as the following:

> "That problem is important. We need to give it the attention it deserves. Let's set up another time when we can really sit down and you can talk more about it. You've done a good job of letting me know of your concerns. This will also give me some time to think things through for you. Does that sound like a good plan?"

The wise advisor confirms the most important issue by stating it out loud – for example, "So the number one issue for you right now is how Nora will be deciding where she wants to go to college, am I right?" When the client affirms aloud that this is the main issue, the advisor and the advisee establish a contract. The advisor can refer to this contract throughout the conversation to respectfully refocus the talk if it starts to become tangential. The advisor might say "That also sounds like an important issue. At the same time, I want to make sure you get a chance to talk about what you said is your number one concern – how Nora will be deciding where she'd like to go to college."

Having a contract for the talk helps the advisor and client to stay patient and calm. Without it, even the most patient advisor can become frustrated, and that irritation can diminish rapport.

Ending the conversation

These talks do not have to be lengthy to be effective. The quality of the advising experience does not necessarily improve with time expansion. Most clients consider an advisor who listens and provides counsel as an unexpected gift. For this reason, clients are often unusually attentive to advisors. Just a few moments of high-quality, careful listening pays off. It actually gives the client the pleasant impression that the time together has been longer than it actually was. When an advisor develops good rapport, and the client gets into a comfortable flow of conversation, something interesting often happens. The advisor and the client can become so involved, so focused, that they move into a positive, trance-like state and can lose track of time. While that experience can be very healing for the client, the advisor still needs to maintain a sense of time passage to avoid spending more time than is practicable. Like the Olympic gymnast who ends a great vault by sticking the landing, the advisor should do the same,[16] and respectfully end the conversation. And like the Olympic gymnast, the advisor is often judged by a high-quality and well-timed finish. The advisor needs to take the initiative to move the experience out of this trance-like state. By developing an internal clock, the advisor gauges how much time has elapsed. As the time when the conversation needs to end draws closer, the advisor needs to avoid new content areas, because that would just falsely encourage the client to think there is more time. And if the client opens up a new area and it is emotional, there will not be enough time to soothingly bring matters to a calming end.

Advisors benefit from having some closing moves to stick the landing and signal the end of the conversation. If this is a face-to-face meeting, the advisor should sit down for the talk if possible. A seated advisor now has one clear conversation-closing move available, and that is to literally stand up. As appropriate, the advisor can shake hands and use all the other non-verbal parting signals like a closing smile or an exchange of dates for the next talk.

Advisors have also successfully signaled that the conversation is nearing its end by using such remarks as:

> "We are getting close to the end of our conversation today, let me see if I'm with you."
>
> "Excuse me for a moment. I have just a minute or so before I have to go. What you have been saying is so important, I'd be happy to meet with you again if you'd like."
>
> "Wow, I'm sorry. I realize I'm running out of time. Would you like to talk about this again?"
>
> "Excuse me, Bob, I'm afraid that I'm going to have to run in a moment."

There will be times when the advisor will just have to respectfully interrupt the client, offer a direct observation about the time, say goodbye, and then possibly offer to talk again. To achieve this, the advisor may have to talk over the client. Because a good rapport has typically been established and the client appreciates the advisor's listening, this usually works out quite well.

COGNITIVE THERAPY: THINKING CREATES EMOTIONS

An advisor can encourage hope by commenting that regardless of the problem, the client never has to feel stuck. This is because there are always four options available for handling a problem. The advisor would teach the client to ask the following questions:

➤ Can I get away from it? (e.g. by physically removing myself)
➤ Can I let it be? (e.g. by accepting it)
➤ Can I alter it? (e.g. by working on the problem), *or*
➤ Can I detoxify it? (e.g. by thinking about it in a less poisonous way).

The client can remember this as the GLAD approach. The client has already probably taken at least one of these actions, and that is admirable in the midst of whatever stress they have been experiencing. GLAD helps the client to take credit for what they have already tried, and then opens their mind to other empowering options. Introducing GLAD is also a helpful way to approach the important choice to *detoxify* what happened. Here is a scenario of how a woman client processed GLAD, which led her to decide to include working on detoxifying her problem.

> "Get away from it? I've thought about this for almost eight years now. If I try real hard and, despite my best effort, there is no real change, I'll get a divorce. I'd hate to do it but it's an option I have to consider if it came to that. Look, I have a lot of years ahead of me. I do not want to live them in a loveless marriage."

"**L**et it be? I actually tried that for years. I've seen people who seem to have a marriage like mine. They look like they've learned how to accept it. It seems to work out OK for them. But you know, I really have already tried that approach for years. It wouldn't work for me. Certainly not in the long run. Life is just too short for me to have to settle."

"**A**lter it? Well, do you mean could I try other ways to improve my marriage? Well, I suppose I could re-group one more time and really put my heart into fixing my marriage. Maybe we could finally go for marriage therapy. I could talk to my husband about that. I think he'd agree. He's clearly not happy either. We can look for a psychologist who can see both sides. It could really help."

"**D**etoxify it? Well, if you mean not making as big a deal about this as I have been, I'm not so sure. The truth is, it is bad. It's hard not to think of this as a terrible tragedy. But I think I see what you're suggesting. You're saying to not let my thoughts about it get out of proportion, right? You're right. I'm sure that way of thinking doesn't help me. I'll try and rein that in a bit."

The advisor can close this talk by commenting on how impressively the client used GLAD, and confirm where the client has arrived with her decision making:

"So, it sounds like you are ruling out two options: **G**et away from it and **L**et it be. You are going ahead with the other two GLAD options: **A**lter it, by talking to your husband about marital counseling, and **D**etoxify it, by avoiding discouraging language."

"I'm sorry for all the trouble you've been experiencing in your marriage for so long. At the same time, I'm really impressed with how you thought things through. I would be happy to talk with you about an approach called cognitive therapy. It is all about detoxifying what has been going on so you can be even more clearheaded as you work on altering it through the marriage counseling."

The most widely research-validated of all the psychotherapies is cognitive therapy, also known as rational-emotive therapy, which was developed by Ellis.[17,18] The organizing principle in cognitive therapy is that toxic feelings such as road rage, for example, are determined not by the unpleasant event itself (e.g. a major traffic jam), but by the toxic, irrational thoughts that clients project onto that event. In this context, irrational means rigid, inflexible, illogical, unempirical, or unhelpful. These beliefs are characterized by dogmatic and absolutist demands that clients put on themselves. This includes all the shoulds, musts, have tos, and got tos which lead clients to illogical conclusions such as "I am worthless", "It's awful", or "I can't stand it."

These core assumptions can be summarized in the A-B-C-D-E framework that forms the cornerstone of cognitive therapy interventions. The Activating event triggers evaluative Beliefs, which then lead to Consequences in clients' emotional, physiological, and behavioral lives.

In cognitive therapy, these mean-spirited evaluative beliefs are Disputed vigorously, and replaced with more rational, helpful, and truthful beliefs, resulting in healthier Emotions and constructive behaviors.[19] The cornerstone of this approach is that events do not cause toxic feelings. Toxic feelings are caused by clients' toxic, negative, untrue, and self-critical thoughts about those events. Clients are so well practiced in this habit that they are often unaware that they are doing this.

The role of the advisor is to help clients to:
➤ identify events that trigger negative thoughts
➤ notice the extremely negative and untrue spin that they put on these thoughts, *and*
➤ commit to vigorously put healthy thoughts in place of the unhealthy thoughts.

Clients need to hear from the advisor that feeling emotions is very healthy. Emotions give clients the fuel to act in their best interest. Navigating a car through a major traffic jam can set up a client to feel upset. This is a healthy feeling. It nudges the client to focus, become more alert, and possibly adjust their speed to avoid bumping into the car directly in front. However, the clients who may take this to the road rage level would perceive this traffic jam in extremely negative, absolute, impractical, and untrue terms by quickly thinking "This is the last straw", "This is a catastrophe", "This is terrible", "I can't stand this anymore", "This should not happen", "This must not happen", "I can't believe this is happening", or "This always happens to me." When the advisor can help clients to really understand the meaning of this language and their role in setting up toxic feelings, it becomes clear that these are also just untrue statements. The truth is that it is not the last straw, catastrophes are more monumental events than this traffic jam, the word "terrible" comes from the word "terror", and it is just unhelpful for clients to tell themselves that something should or must not happen when it already has happened. Using these catastrophic, extremely negative descriptors takes its toll. In a sense, the brain begins to believe what it is told.

Carrying around these kinds of negative thoughts is like carrying around a harsh critic or bully in the brain. Clients can emotionally drown in these feelings, unable to think clearly. That is, for example, where road rage can originate. When negative and exaggerated thoughts highjack people's emotions, this causes some individuals to make poor choices (e.g. dangerously chasing down that reckless driver).

The advisor can talk to clients about not entertaining such toxic and untrue thoughts. Yet it is a challenge to *not* think about something. The advisor can ask the client to try not to think of the color red. It's not easy. It is easier not to think of the color red by thinking of a different color instead. For example, "Think of the color blue." This holds for negative thinking as well. In place of the negative thoughts, the advisor can suggest the following three-part sequence:

1 "**It would be better if** . . . there was not a major traffic jam this morning" (this is said in a more casual tone of voice).
2 "**But the truth is** . . . there is a major traffic jam this morning" (this is said in a more matter-of-fact, objective tone of voice).
3 "**And** it's not a catastrophe . . . in fact I must be a pretty good driver the way I am avoiding bumping into other cars" (this is said in a more energized, determined, and powerful tone of voice).

Note that three different tones of voice are used here. This is because merely reciting the corrective statements to oneself in a calm way may be insufficient to combat a powerfully over-learned habit. The advisor can suggest that the client practices the sequence using the demeanor and tone of a very assertive person or a television or movie character, and to use that powerful attitude which is so important in combating these discouraging perceptions.

Here is another example of this same approach used by a 13-year-old, middle-school-aged student who is being verbally bullied by a classmate.[20]

1 "**It would be better** if . . . Todd didn't give me a rough time" (this is said in a more casual tone of voice).
2 "**But the truth is** . . . Todd does give me a rough time" (this is said in a more matter-of-fact, objective tone of voice).
3 "**And** I can stand it" or "**And** I refuse to let this get to me like it used to" or "**And** this is not good, for sure, but it is not a catastrophe!" or "**And** I'm not going to put myself down like I used to" (this is said in a more energized, determined, and powerful tone of voice).

There is another cognitive approach that challenges two client misconceptions. It combats the tendency to over-exaggerate the likelihood that something bad will happen. It also combats the tendency that, in the very unlikely event that the bad thing did happen, the client could not handle it. Here is an example. Kristine has received excellent reviews from her work supervisor, Patrick, for the last four years. Because Patrick did not say hello to her while passing in the hall-way, Kristine is getting worried that this means he is planning to reprimand her. The advisor can suggest that Kristine should ask herself the following two ques-tions which will reduce the distorted thinking:

➤ *Question 1*: "**What is the evidence that this** ('my supervisor is planning to reprimand me') **is going to happen?**"

Answer: "This is a very low likelihood situation. Frankly, there is no evidence that this would happen. Patrick has been a big supporter of my work. He's probably just thinking about his own direct responsibilities. C'mon, I have had great reviews from him. Knock it off, these are silly thoughts. Just last week Patrick gave me a compliment. I need to think about what a good job I've been doing."

➤ *Question 2*: "**In the rare likelihood that this did happen, what is the evidence that I could not handle it?**"

Answer: "There is no evidence that I couldn't handle it. Again, it's not likely at all that I will be reprimanded. But if I was, I'd just ask Patrick what I can do to make it better. Besides, I have handled much tougher situations than that in my life."

In summary, the advisor can help clients to begin to talk sense to themselves when confronted with life's triggers, and also to challenge themselves to search for the evidence that an undesired event is going to happen, and if it did that they couldn't handle it.

SOCIAL PROBLEM SOLVING: HELPING CLIENTS TO RESOLVE THEIR OWN DIFFICULTIES

There are times when clients want the advisor to supply them with facts and answers. This works well when the advisor knows that particular problem con-tent area. For the many occasions when the advisor is not the content expert, a significant expansion of the role is called for. The advisor needs to move from being a solver of the client's problem to being a facilitator of the client's problem-solving thinking. Clients are more likely anyway to use the ideas that they thought of, rather than those of someone else. When clients witness their own problem-solving thinking, their self-esteem rises and they feel empowered. To be skilled in this powerful approach, the advisor can use a roadmap. A social problem-solving roadmap helps the advisor to avoid feeling pressured to supply all the answers, and also protects the advisor from getting lost in the details and emotions of the troubling story.

Social problem solving (SPS), sometimes referred to as problem-solving therapy, teaches a strategy for thinking clearly and in a step-wise fashion to confidently confront challenging situations. Social problem solving was originally proposed by D'Zurilla and Goldfried,[21] and was subsequently adapted over the years as a school-based intervention and problem prevention strategy for children,[22] and cultivated as a psychotherapy.[23]

A meta-analysis of 32 randomized controlled trials in which SPS was applied to a wide range of emotional and physical problems concluded that such a problem-solving therapy was as effective as other psychosocial treatments, and significantly superior to attention placebo or no treatment conditions.[24] Another meta-analysis of 13 randomized controlled trials[25] found that problem-solving therapy is clearly an effective treatment for depression. In one study, practitioners in family medicine and primary care offices either provided patients who had minor depression with a six-step social problem-solving intervention, or offered a usual care treatment of watchful waiting, treatment with antidepressant medications, brief supportive counseling, or external referral to a mental health provider. At both the 4-week and 6-month follow-up, patients in all of the treatment conditions showed improvement. However, patients who were treated with the social problem-solving intervention had a faster rate of improvement in depressive symptoms than participants in the other interventions. In a review of psychosocial interventions delivered by general practitioners,[26] problem-solving treatment for depression was described as the most promising tool for general practitioners. The application of social problem solving as a clinical intervention has been wide-ranging. For example, one study concluded that social problem solving should be included as an important clinical target to consider in the development of psychological interventions to assist people with non-cardiac chest pain.[27]

When clients without good social problem-solving skills are highly stressed, they can become so flooded with feelings that they have difficulty generating goal-directed, alternative solutions to their problem. This deficit causes them to feel helpless and hopeless. When this happens chronically, it can understandably lead to depression.[28]

The advisor can use the following roadmap from the social problem-solving tradition: Problem, Emotion, Goal, and Solutions (also known as PEGS). The advisor facilitates the flow of the talk in the following direction:

1 Problem: Tell me what the problem is.
2 Emotions: How do you feel about that?

3   Goal: What do you want to have happen?
4   Solutions: Think of as many solutions to the problem as you can.

The PEGS concept emerges from social problem solving (SPS) which takes a problem prevention approach as well as a psychotherapeutic one.

Here is a case example of how SPS works. Dr. Schottland is a family physician who is in the role of an advisor for his patient Sheila, a high school junior. Dr. Schottland uses PEGS as a roadmap to guide his conversation with Sheila.

Problem

Dr. Schottland: "Sheila, what's the problem?"

Sheila: "My soccer coach turned on me at the end of last season. She started doing a lot of name calling and would insult me all practice long. I think she likes getting on my case. I don't know if I really want to play anymore."

Naming the problem brings cognitive clarity. By asking Sheila to narrow down her description into a problem statement, Dr. Schottland transforms a cloudy, confusing situation into a potentially more manageable issue.

Emotions

Dr. Schottland: "How do you feel?"

Sheila: "I want to quit."

Dr. Schottland: "I hear you. How do you feel about this?"

Sheila: "I don't know. I've been better. I'm a little out of it lately . . . kind of disappointed I guess."

Giving Sheila an opportunity to describe her inner life is quite therapeutic. Notice how the advisor did not back off when Sheila did not initially say how she felt. The simple act of Sheila naming how she feels provides clarity for her. Like many of us, she may be struggling with multiple confusing emotions. Naming her feelings also gives Sheila a much better chance of clearly explaining herself to others. These others, like Dr. Schottland, Sheila's friends, or her parents might now be able to understand and maybe support her, validate her, and help out.

Goal

Dr. Schottland: "What is your goal? What do you want to have happen?"

Sheila: "I want to make it harder for her to insult me."

Here Dr. Schottland focuses on helping Sheila to set a reasonable and reach-able goal. The doctor wants to encourage Sheila's ambition and energy and at the same time guide her toward that goal. For instance, Sheila might have ini-tially said that her goal was to get the coach to stop insulting her. This kind of goal statement can be a challenge for advisors. For example, people who are prone to depression often set themselves up for disappointment with unrealis-tic goals. Sheila is headed for more frustration if her goal is to change someone else's behavior. In the role of advisor, Dr. Schottland would coach and guide her to modify that goal from a likely frustrating one to a more reachable one. Unlike Don Quixote, people need to dream a more possible dream as a way to start feeling empowered. They can then move on to a gradually more challeng-ing dream if they wish.

The advisor who has authentically and consistently been empathetic will be able to suggest re-formulating the goal. The advisor's first step should be to gently validate and empathize with Sheila's desire "to get Coach to stop insult-ing me." Dr. Schottland can say "It makes sense that you would want a goal like getting Coach off your back. At the same time I'm concerned. A goal to change another person is tough to expect of yourself. I can't blame you for wanting that, but it's a rough one to expect of yourself. What's another goal that you have a good chance of delivering on?" If Sheila struggles to come up with a new goal, Dr. Schottland can suggest one. In this case maybe a more reachable goal could be something like "to make it more difficult for Coach to insult me."

Solutions

Dr. Schottland: "What are all the possible solutions that could help you get there?"

Sheila: "I could start coming to practice earlier than anyone else and even stay later to show I'm motivated."

"Our assistant coach is actually one of my biggest fans. I could tell her, but that would make it worse, because I'd look disloyal."

"I could just tell Coach what I think about the way she has been treating me."

When Sheila has started to generate her solutions, she can begin to perceive herself as a problem solver. She no longer has to feel stuck or that there is no way out of social problems. In more extreme examples, such as with depressed patients who have suicidal thoughts, social problem-solving techniques like PEGS could save a life.

Poor social problem solvers respond to a tough problem by becoming over-whelmed or even panicking. However, good social problem solvers see the onset of a problem as a cue to problem solve. PEGS can be one of Sheila's tools that she can rely on. Clients who learn a four-step social problem-solving approach such as PEGS tend to adopt some personally meaningful aspect(s) of this clear thinking strategy and make it their own. For Sheila it might be to remember that there is always more than one way to solve a problem. For another client, it might be to remember always to have a goal in mind. For others it might be to establish a goal and generate solutions. What will Sheila absorb from these brief conversations with Dr. Schottland? One day when she may most need it, Sheila may say to herself, "I remember once my doctor telling me that I don't have to feel trapped by problems." Again, this could save an impulsive, depressed client's life.

SOLUTION-FOCUSED ADVISING: FROM MISERY TALK TO POSITIVE TALK

Some people seem to be stuck in misery talk. Talking about how miserable things are seems to perpetuate more misery talk. It discourages the creative thinking that generates solutions, and it robs people of happiness. Solution-focused advising comes from the *solution-oriented therapy* tradition,[29] in which the advisor guides troubled people to think about what they are doing, thinking, and feeling during times when they are feeling better. The content of the conversation anticipates a more positive future and creates hope.

The advisor does not directly teach skills. Instead, they ask the client about the exceptions to the client's problem, and to look at what happens when the problem is less intense or has gone. The conversation moves away from the problem-soaked present and past, and towards a solution-focused future.[30] This focus on exceptions was a distinguishing feature of work done by Steve de Shazer, Insoo Kim Berg and their colleagues at the Family Therapy Center in Milwaukee.[31]

Solution-oriented psychotherapy represents unique challenges for evaluation, and so it is at the early stages of formal research regarding its efficacy.[32] In solution-oriented psychotherapy, things move very quickly. The intervention begins at the assessment stage. Because most outcome measures are problem-focused in nature, it is difficult to gather pre- and post-intervention assessments in the solution-oriented approach. As the client is explaining the current misery, the advisor is already making changes therapeutically. Solution-oriented approaches shift the discussion almost immediately to strengths. A good summary of the obstacles to research in this area comes from a patient who completed several depression and symptom inventories and who said "I thought I was doing all right until I had to fill out those forms."[33] Despite these challenges, there remains a growing effort to evaluate solution-oriented psychotherapy. And although there is not yet a strong evidence base,[34] in the view of this author (JC) it is clearly a promising practice. Of ten studies that were recently reviewed,[35] four were rated as having a moderate to high effect size and, in psychotherapy outcome, even a small effect size might show an important result.[36] Therefore about 50% of the studies of solution-oriented psychotherapy show improvement over other conditions or no-treatment controls.[37] Because of its promise, several of the key techniques of solution-oriented psychotherapy are offered here.

The following is a case example of solution-focused advising. Joan is 31 years old, married, with no children, and commutes to a full-time job in the city as a loan officer in a bank. She is depressed but not suicidal. She says to the advisor "I'm dealing with a lot of sadness and loss. My parents divorced when I was 19 and I just never got over that. My mother died a few years ago. I feel guilty that I never did enough to get her the care she needed. I'm overweight and out of shape. And now I'm drinking with my husband two or three drinks at night just to relax and unwind. That's not good either. I'm just depressed."

In solution-focused advising,[38] the focus is on the positive, the solution, the patient's strengths, and the future. The content of the conversation is on solution talk rather than on problem talk. There are essentially four parts to the advisor's strategy:

1 **Empathize.**
2 **Find out what the client is doing, thinking, or feeling during those times when things are going better.**
3 **Deepen the understanding of what exactly the client is doing when things are going better.**
4 **Ask what steps the client could take to get on track to getting closer to doing those things.**

In this example, the advisor would empathize with Joan and then ask "When are these problems not happening? And what are you doing during that time?" This approach challenges Joan to consider that things are probably not all bad all the time. As she reflects on how she is behaving when things are better, she can then begin to take small steps to get closer to that desired state. She will feel more in charge of her life.

These are the ten simple assumptions of solution-focused advising:

1 There are **advantages to a positive focus**. By moving the focus to the positive, to solutions, to the person's strengths, and to the future, the advisor facilitates a shift towards the desired direction.

2 The **exceptions to the pain will suggest solutions**. Exceptions to every problem can be created. These exceptions are used to build solutions. The advisor would ask "What is going on during those times when you are not depressed?"

3 **Nothing is always the same.** In fact, change occurs all the time. Even a client who is feeling depressed acts at times in ways that lessen the depression. And saying that a client is depressed is confining and limiting. The meaning is quite different from stating that a client acts depressed.

4 **Small changes often lead to bigger changes.** If a client makes a positive change in one aspect of life, there will be a positive connection to another area. For example, the fact that Joan has started to take brief walks in the evening to raise her mood can inspire her to also reduce her alcohol consumption in the evening.

5 **Cooperation is inevitable.** Clients show how they think change takes place for them. It is important to pay attention to and honor that. In this way, clients can be seen as always cooperating. Many advisors incorrectly pick the problem that they think should be worked on. For example, an advisor may try to push Joan to reduce her alcohol consumption as a first priority. However, Joan may see it differently and want to start with walking or exercise. An advisor who understands and works with Joan's priorities will attract greater cooperation.

6 **Clients are resourceful.** They have all that they need to solve their problems. Joan has graduated from college, left home to create her own household, did this with another person, and has a job. These are significant accomplishments involving considerable problem solving, resourcefulness, and energy. The advisor should respect this and help Joan to do the same.

7 **The client is the expert.** In solution-focused advising, the idea is that no one knows Joan, and what would work best for her, better than herself.

8 **If it's not broken, don't fix it.** An advisor may notice something of concern but the client does not. Unless it is a dangerous situation, the advisor should avoid going there and focus on what the client has stated is the number one issue.

9 The advisor should **handle each talk as if it were the last and only time they will see that client**. This will heighten the advisor's focus.

10 If the advisor's task or question has not seemed to work, this does not mean that the advisor is a failure. The client's response is only feedback, and is merely a signal for the advisor to try something different.

Goals that change behavior

An advisor makes it easier for a client to change by co-crafting goals with the following characteristics.[39]

Phrase the goal in a positive way

It is about what the client will be doing or thinking, rather than what they will *not* be doing or thinking.

Advisor:	"Joan, in place of the two drinks you and your husband are having in the evening, what will you be doing instead?"
Joan:	"I'd probably start eating more sensibly, maybe even getting to bed at a reasonable time."

Storyboard the goal

The advisor should help the client to storyboard the goal the way a movie director does when setting up a scene for the actors. This evokes powerful change-oriented action. Here is how advisors can phrase this.

Advisor:	"Joan, how will you be eating more sensibly?"
Joan:	"Well, I suppose I would be eating smaller portions and having smaller meals and doing this more frequently."

When the client can describe what would literally be happening and discussed, this is creating a powerful goal.

Start today

The client should start working on the solution immediately. The goal therefore needs to be described in present-day terms. Unfortunately, many clients treat their goals as if they were targets in the distant future. The advisor needs to intervene here. For example:

Joan:	"I want to make a decision as to whether to start exercising at home or in a class." This goal is too far in the future and too removed for the client to feel any control. The goal should be defined in an active way, where the client can get on track immediately.
Advisor:	"Joan, as you leave here today, and you are on track to making a decision, what will you be doing differently or saying differently to yourself?"

Joan:	"I'll probably find out about where I can take a group exercise class . . . I'm better off exercising with at least one other person."

Ask for specifics

Advisor:	"How specifically will you be doing this?"
Joan:	"I'll talk to my husband tonight about changing our routine at home, not watching TV as much and not having drinks. We could walk together and say hello to our neighbors."

It is the client who should take action, not someone else.

This criterion is critical. Many clients complain that they want someone else to change or be different. This is often an endless and fruitless effort. A quality goal is one that clients can start on and maintain by themselves.

Joan:	"I want my husband to start living a more healthy life."
Advisor:	"For sure, that would be great. What could you do to get that going, Joan?"
Joan:	"I'll probably be the one suggesting the walk. You know, maybe I'll make us a fruit smoothie in a nice cocktail glass, rather than something alcoholic."

Remembering times when the problem had disappeared or the goal was reached

Here are two examples of how an advisor can move the client away from misery talk and towards solution talk. In this case, Clay is a 45-year-old married accountant with three children under the age of 10 years.

Clay:	"I don't really get along with my wife anymore. I get really cranky and irritable with her and the kids. I wish my wife would understand me better and we didn't fight so much about the kids and money."
Advisor:	"Clay, what is your main goal? What is the most important thing you want to accomplish?"
Clay:	"To start acting more calmly."
Advisor:	"OK, that's really clear. Tell me about the times when you act a little that way now."
Clay:	"This may sound weird, but I think I'm calmer when I have a better handle on our finances. I'd like to know exactly where our money goes each month. I think I need a budget."

Here is the second example of an advisor helping the client to move in a positive direction by offering an exception-oriented question or statement.

Clay: "I hate being so cranky with everyone at home."

Advisor: "Clay, when doesn't the problem happen?"

Clay: "Well, that's a hard one. Actually, it seems that when I'm in a regular exercise routine it helps. To be honest, it's also when I've cut back on the beers . . ."

There are other methods that can also activate positive thinking.

First, hypotheticals can help. If the client cannot recall occasions when the goal was reached or the problem was reduced, the advisor should respect this and then ask about a hypothetical solution. Here is an example:

Advisor: "Clay, it sounds like it's hard coming up with examples of when things are better currently. Let's change this a bit. Imagine a time in the future when things are going better for you. With that in mind, and you were on track to getting along with your wife better, what would you be doing differently?"

Clay: "I'd have that budget. I probably also would have a schedule of the kids' activities and where they need to be. If I had that, there'd be less last-minute hustling to figure out who has to drive which one where. I probably would be getting a family calendar together and keeping it updated."

The second method involves looking at what another person would observe. To uncork a client's stuck thinking, the advisor asks the client to imagine what another person would observe if things were going well. The question is simply "If someone else saw you doing well, what would that person observe?"

Advisor: "Clay, let's imagine for a moment that you were getting along in a calm and pleasant way with your wife. What would another person, looking on, see you doing differently?"

Clay: "Probably that person would see me not being so nasty and insulting her point of view."

Advisor: "What would this person see you doing instead?"

Clay: "Probably I'd be letting my wife finish what she had to say before stating my opinion, and I'd be using more polite language."

While hypotheticals can be helpful, the real-life recall of when things are actually better is often a more powerful approach. For example, there are times when a client enters the revolving door of a building, encounters the door at a dead stop and needs to push the door from this dead stop. The client has to overcome all of this inertia. However, if the client comes to the door as someone is leaving and the door is still moving, this is much easier.[40] This is true about making a behavior or attitude change as well. If the client can see the goal as continuing what he or she has already begun doing, the inertia does not exist. The client only has to keep the door moving. Real-life exceptions put the solution in the realm of the possible and the present. The present is a much more compelling time than the remote past or the far distant future.

In summary, there are seven steps to solution-oriented advising.

1 Listen, paraphrase, and empathize.
2 Move the client from misery talk to solution talk with such invitations as "Tell me about when you are already doing some of what you want", "Tell me about when the problem is not happening", or "If others were observing you when you were feeling better, how would they describe what you are doing?"
3 Elicit the context by asking "What is going on that is different about these times?"
4 Storyboard these ideas by suggesting "Let's imagine that we were making a movie scene of what you are doing differently during that time" and asking "What would you specifically be doing or perhaps even thinking differently in that movie scene?"
5 Reinforce and deepen the change by making such inquiries as "How did you decide to do that?" and "How do you explain that?", and by affirming "That (name the behavior) is really great!"
6 Create achievable, positive expectations by commenting "So, after our conversation today, what would be the signs that you were continuing to get yourself on track?"
7 Maintain change by asking "What steps do you see yourself taking to keep this going?"

MOTIVATIONAL ADVISING: ACTIONS SPEAK LOUDER THAN WORDS

Motivational advising is when the advisor discovers the client's exciting dreams and then uses those dreams as a springboard to help the client to change behavioral habits in order to achieve them. It is about facilitating a client's own incentive to change.

Eating more sensibly, stopping nicotine use, changing a relationship with alcohol, exercising, flossing, and taking vitamins and medicines as prescribed are all great examples of health habits that can be adopted and solidified. Young children often make the changes that trusted adults (e.g. parent figures, teachers, physicians) suggest. They tend not to question. However, adult clients are different. They are seasoned with their own success and failures and have formed their own perspectives as appropriate. Clients do not make changes in their personal lives just because someone in authority recommends it. Simply put, clients want the advisor to ask about and respect their experience. Clients prefer that the advisor does not pound them with factual information, much of which they may already know (e.g. the dangers of smoking, drinking excessively, or eating fast foods). Some clients, out of annoyance and pride, may react to an advisor's pontificating in a way that entrenches the unhealthy behavior pattern. Clients change when they are emotionally energized to do so. Change is more about the heat than the light.

In *motivational interviewing (MI)*, the advisor elicits and strengthens the client's motivation to change, and evokes real behavior change in the face of ambivalence. While many clients fully understand that making a behavioral change is in their best interest, they are simultaneously aware that this will also cost them something. It is this ambivalence that may influence them to make only a half-hearted change, or not to make any change at all.[41] It is best to think about MI as a form of communication where the advisor elicits the client's motivation to change and makes it easier for the client to reach their goal. The advisor and the client are on the same team. MI does not force change from the unwilling client, nor is it a cognitive-behavioral therapy (CBT) type of skill teaching. MI helps clients to develop, articulate, and deepen their own arguments for change.[42] It is rare that clients would argue with their own argument! Pascal is quoted as saying "People are generally better persuaded by the reasons which they themselves have discovered than by those which have come into the minds of others."[43]

A meta-analysis[44] of 72 published clinical trials of MI indicated that while the strongest scientific support was in the area of substance abuse, there was also support for its use in other behavior change-challenging areas, such as adhering to treatment, dieting, exercising, HIV risk reduction efforts, and other health safety practices. The conclusion of another meta-analysis[45] was that motivational interviewing is superior to traditional advice-giving in assisting people with a wide range of diseases and behavioral problems. With 30 years of studies to support it, motivational interviewing has been shown to be evidence based, relatively brief, applicable to a wide range of problem areas, a useful adjunct to all kinds of advising approaches, and easily learnable by a wide variety of advisors who want to help others.[46] With unhealthy behaviors, emotions often supersede reason. Clients make behavioral decisions that appear to be irrational.[47] They frequently decide that the short-term emotional benefits (e.g. "Smoking helps me to relax") are more important than the long-term quantifiable benefits (e.g. "to live better and longer").

Clients approach advisors for help because they regard advisors as people who have had significant success in fixing problems. Unfortunately, being good at fixing problems for others plays a limited role in facilitating behavior change. In the medical field, for example, directive advice about behavior change works with only a minority of patients, and can sometimes have the opposite effect. Most advisors can recall being teenagers and being told not to do something by parents, which actually led to the opposite effect. Directive messages such as "You should . . . or else . . ." often prove counterproductive.[48] The wise saying that nothing is as practical as a theory is particularly true in motivational interviewing. The advisor must understand where a client may be on the "readiness to change" continuum before determining what to say to promote healthy behavior. The classic source for this model is the *five stages of change*,[49] which was developed from smoking cessation research. The stages can be summarized as follows.

➤ Stage 1: **Pre-contemplation ("No way")**. When asked if there is an interest in changing, this is the client who says "No way." There is not even a contemplation of change. It is hard to get any more negative than this! There is no interest in even discussing taking the medicines as prescribed, improving the diet, or improving parenting skills. When advising people at Stage 1, advisors have to be careful of their own zealousness. If advisors insist on pushing their own point of view, the client could become irritated and directly make this known in word, action, and tone. Or the client could give the advisor what might appear to be an agreement, but is actually a politely disguised resentment laid over some passive aggressiveness and an inclination to become even more set in the bad habit. One of the best ways to handle a pre-contemplator is to respectfully paraphrase the client's decision and then show availability when the client is ready to make the healthy change. For example, the advisor might say "Sounds like now is not the right time for you to make that change. When you are ready, let me know and I'll be glad to help", and then gracefully move on to another topic. This will help to keep the relationship intact for future talks when the client is indeed contemplating change.

➤ Stage 2: **Contemplation ("Maybe")**. Here there is a little movement, as the client is actually contemplating the possibility of changing. A client at this stage usually expresses ambivalence about change: "I'm not really sure about starting to exercise. I've never considered myself an athlete, I used to try and get out of physical education in school as much as I could. I just don't know." Here the advisor asks about the client's intermediate and long-term goals, with questions such as "If things go well for you, what do you look forward to doing?" Using this thoughtful approach, the advisor can help a client who is at this stage to explore the advantages and disadvantages of, for example, not exercising. Then the advisor asks the client to make a decision about a behavior change. It is a non-lecturing approach to facilitate progress toward greater well-being.

➤ Stage 3: **Preparation ("OK").** The client who is at this stage is ready to change and is ready to begin the important business of planning. This client may perhaps be selecting a date to begin exercise, buying comfortable athletic shoes, arranging with others to take walks after dinner, and so on.

➤ Stage 4: **Action ("Do it").** Here the client is actually starting to change. Perhaps the client is actually putting on the athletic shoes and walking outside after dinner.

➤ Stage 5: **Maintenance ("Keep it going").** The client at this stage is determined to make the change a lasting habit. There is a commitment, for example, whether it is raining or not, to take a walk every day. The after-dinner walk becomes such a routine that the client's neighbors would notice if the routine changed slightly.

Guidelines for changing behavioral habits with motivational advising

Express empathy for the problem as well as the challenge of changing

The advisor should express an understanding of and empathy for a person's plight (e.g. "That's difficult, to feel stuck in a job that really does not match your interests"). If they feel understood, the client will be less likely to continue to provide public testimony about how hard it would be to change. They no longer have to repeat the feelings of stuckness, thus entrenching the negative habit.

It is also strategically critical to provide high-quality empathy about how difficult changing might be for the client (e.g. "At the same time, it is challenging to think about how to find a new job"). The advisor should remember that behavioral change is more about emotion than about logic. So reflecting back the client's feelings and experience helps the client to fully experience the dilemma,[50] which will in turn help them to leave it.

Most questions should tap arguments for change

This is one of the most important concepts and interventions of motivational advising. As has already been mentioned, the talking out loud by the client about what makes it so difficult to find a new job, avoid fried foods, or stop smoking or drinking may actually reinforce the paralysis. Asking questions about the obstacles to change or what gets in the way of change tends to entrench the behavior pattern. The advisor should avoid asking "What makes it so difficult to find a new job in your field?", and instead should ask "When people successfully make career changes in your field, how do they go about doing it?" The advisor should remember to begin with authentically empathizing. It will then be much easier to help the client to move over to some positive talk. The wise advisor should think, think, and think again about the formulation of questions, and only ask the questions that, when answered, pull for positive change talk.

Avoid argumentation

Arguments reinforce defensiveness. A client might say "But you just don't understand, putting a good résumé together is a lot of work, and it takes a lot of time." If the advisor counters with a comment like "Well, it really does not have to take up that much time", they may technically be correct. However, motivational advising is not about the advisor being correct. Meeting a person's resistance with a contrary and factually correct point of view, as well-meaning as it is intended, pushes the client to escalate and defend, by saying, for example, "Well, in my field you wouldn't believe what has to go into a really good résumé." Or the client may become silently resentful or withdraw. Instead, the advisor should join the resistance by acknowledging the client's frustration and thus removing this as an argument point. The client's energy can thus be saved and put to better use in pursuing healthy change.

The advisor and client competing on the same team

Motivational advising elicits the discrepancies and competition that are healthy. An unhealthy form of competition would be that between what the client does (e.g. smoking) and what the advisor prefers that the client would do (e.g. not smoking). Competition within the team should be avoided. The advisor who helps a client to move towards healthy habits develops a healthier competition, where the client and the advisor are on the same team. The competition is then between the advisor/client team and the obstacles to the client's healthy goal.

Other forms of healthy competition in motivational advising could be between the positive aspects of the present behavior and the positive aspects of the new behavior, or between the negative aspects of the current behavior and the negative aspects of the new behavior. The advisor should make the discrepancy be about the client's current behavior and their life goal. For example, the advisor could ask what the client is looking forward to doing one day. The client may reveal that they want to cycle with family members. The advisor asks for more encouraging details about that goal, pauses, and then creates a healthy therapeutic doubt by commenting "That is a wonderful goal. I can see you doing that, cycling with your family and having such fun. I'm not sure how continuing smoking will help you get there."

The advisor then pauses. This allows for a moment of awkward and yet therapeutic silence. The client can reflect for a moment. The advisor can then ask what the client has decided to do about the current behavior. If the decision is to make a healthy change, the advisor and the client can work together as a formidable team to get the client to a state of some day going cycling with the family.

Support positive expectations

In the psychological literature, this is also known as self-efficacy. It is key to motivational advising as well as to any other model that explains how people change. The client needs to believe that:

1 it is important to change
2 the advisor's advice will help
3 the advice is implementable.

Respect the incentive of impulsive people

Clients who eat a lot of fatty foods at fast food restaurants, or who would rather watch a television comedy than exercise, could be considered impulsive. A rational appeal regarding the long-term benefits of changing, or a warning about the long-term impact of not changing, may not work. An alternative strategy is to recognize these impulsive clients as pleasure-seeking. Accordingly, the focus should shift away from the pain of not changing to the pleasure that they would experience if they did change. The advisor might say "Sounds like eating healthy food and exercising will start removing the physical pain. It will give you the physical comfort that comes with freedom of movement. You'll actually be feeling more pleasure."

Use a collaborative and friendly style

An outstanding motivational conversation actually resembles two friends looking at vacation photographs together. One person is telling the story about the vacation. The other person is genuinely curious, listens respectfully, and at times asks some good questions. This listener is friendly and shows personal interest. They want to understand and learn. It is a polite and collaborative exchange. Both people feel good after the conversation and would want to come back and talk again.

Protocol for motivational advising: For the contemplation stage (Maybe)

Here are the steps for using motivational advising with a client who is undecided and still contemplating changing. The advisor should clarify the issue about which there is ambivalence by saying, for example, "So you're not sure about whether to continue your relationship with Frank, even though he sees other women too", and suggest a five- to ten-minute conversation to help. When the time comes, the advisor would begin with the following contract: "For the next ten minutes, perhaps we can go through some questions to help you decide what you'd like to do."

1 Sincerely **inquire about the positive aspects of the behavior**. Clients who rarely have an opportunity to talk about this will often experience some relief. For physicians, it has been said that "Patients become more willing to change if you acknowledge their choice to behave in 'unhealthy' ways and if they think that you really understand their reasons to stay the same."[51] The advisor should use such questions as "What are some of the good things about going out with Frank?"

2 Actively listen, and **summarize** the positive aspects periodically: "It sounds like when you are with Frank he makes you laugh, you like the physical intimacy, he's easy to talk to, and you have made some exciting trips together."

3 **Ask about the negative aspects.** "What are some of the less good things about your seeing Frank?"

4 Actively listen and periodically **summarize** these: "So while you have a good time with Frank, he is not interested in spending time with your son Mike, sometimes he drinks too much and insists on driving, and you are not really too sure about how steady his job is."

5 **Summarize both the positive and negative aspects:** "On the one hand, you're saying that you like Frank's humor, the intimacy, your conversations,

and adventures. On the other hand, he's not interested in Mike, he drives when he has been drinking, and his job may not be stable. Have I understood you so far? Is there anything I missed?"

6 **Solicit the client's life goals.** It will be these goals against which the costs and benefits are weighed. To get at this, the advisor asks questions such as "What do your values tell you are important in your life?", "How do you want your family and friends to see you?", or "If things worked out really great for you, what would you be doing in six months' time?" Using the example of ambivalence about seeing Frank, here is what a client could offer: "Well, what's important to me is being with someone who could be a good father figure and role model for Mike. I don't want to sound too shallow, but I want us to be financially secure enough to be able to buy a house and have a yard to enjoy."

7 **Summarize and praise the goals.** In this case, the advisor might say "The stable and happy family life you have described sounds like a great plan for you and Mike."

8 **Articulate the discrepancy and permit some therapeutic silence:** "At the same time (pause), I'm not sure how being with Frank fits in with where you said you want to be in your life." The advisor is quiet for a moment or two, allowing this discrepancy to linger with the client.

9 **Restate the client's decision-making dilemma and then ask what the client has decided to do:** "You wanted to make a decision about whether to stay with Frank or end the relationship and move on. Where are you now with your decision?"

Often the initially ambivalent client decides to make the positive change. The advisor responds to questions, offers support, and gives the client some time and space in which to think. There may be more considerations to discuss and more decisions to be made, such as how to take the next step, or talking to family members about the decision.

  If the client is still not ready to make a decision, the advisor should empathize with the difficulty of ambivalence. The advisor should then ask "What else (such as time or additional information) would help you to come to a decision?" or "Would you be interested in reducing some of the problem while you are making a decision?"

If the client decides against changing, the advisor of course respects this, offers their availability to assist in any way, and expresses confidence in the person's ability to decide.

For the ambivalent client, the following is a summary of the protocol.

1 The advisor suggests taking five to ten minutes to help the client to sort out the concerns about the decision.

2 The advisor asks "What are some of the good things that you like about (the poor behavioral health behavior)?", and then summarizes these positive aspects for the client.

3 The advisor asks "What don't you like about (the poor behavioral health behavior)?", and then summarizes the negative aspects.

4 The advisor asks about the client's aspirations: "If things worked out in the best possible way for you, what would you be doing in six months' time?", and then paraphrases and praises these goals.

5 The advisor suggests a discrepancy: "At the same time, I'm not sure how (the behavior) fits with those plans."

6 The advisor asks for a decision: "You were saying that you wanted to decide whether to continue (the behavior) or change. Where are you now with your decision?"

7 The advisor closes by anticipating what will happen next: "What will be your next or first step now?"

Effective goal-setting is an important feature of behavior change, and with initially ambivalent clients, it is a helpful next step when they decide to change. The SMART (Specific, Meaningful, Assessable, Realistic, Timed) approach to setting a goal can be very helpful. For example, an advisor is working with Jimmy, who has decided to start exercising.

Specific

Advisor:	"What will be your next (first) step?"
Jimmy:	"I think I'll start walking after dinner. Maybe I'll lift weights, too."

Meaningful

Advisor:	"Sounds like you think if you did that, it would make a real difference."
Jimmy:	"Oh yeah, I'd probably walk for about 20 minutes and for me right now that is a huge difference. Work has gotten so busy – I've been closing some important deals and haven't gotten a chance to exercise in a while."

Assessable

Advisor:	"How will you know that the exercise is working for you?"
Jimmy:	"Easy. I'm going to coach soccer for the kids and I have to run around with them. If I'm not out of breath when I do that with them, I'll know I'm fine. If I start lifting weights again I know how much I want to be able to bench."

Realistic

Advisor:	"So with the kids and phone calls to make, that sounds manageable . . . No?"
Jimmy:	"Absolutely. My oldest can come with me. I can make my calls when I get back. Sometimes I can make a few quick calls on my cell while I'm walking. That's no problem."

Timed

Advisor:	"When do you see yourself starting?"
Jimmy:	"I think I'll start tomorrow night."

REFERENCES

Client strengths, advisor–client rapport, and positive expectations

1 Adler J, Underwood A, Bain M. Freud in our midst. *Newsweek* 2006; **147**: 42–9.

2 Weissman M, Verdeli H, Gameroff M *et al*. National survey of psychotherapy training in psychiatry, psychology, and social work. *Archives of General Psychiatry* 2006; **63**: 925–34.

3 Hubble M, Duncan B, Miller S. *The Heart and Soul of Change: what works in therapy.* Washington, DC: American Psychological Association; 1999.

4 Lambert M. Implications of outcomes research for psychotherapy integration. In: Norcross J, Goldfried M, eds. *Handbook of Psychotherapy Integration.* New York: Basic Books; 1992. pp. 94–129.

5 Johansson H, Eklund M. Patients' opinion on what constitutes good psychiatric care. *Scandinavian Journal of Caring Science* 2003; **17**: 339–46.

6 Priebe S, McCabe R. Therapeutic relationships in psychiatry: the basis of therapy or therapy itself? *International Journal of Psychiatry* 2008; **20**: 521–6.

7 Schrank B, Stanghellini G, Slade M. Hope in psychiatry: a review of the literature. *Acta Psychiatrica Scandinavica* 2008; **118**: 421–33.

8 Stuart M, Lieberman J. *The Fifteen Minute Hour: therapeutic talk in primary care.* 3rd edn. Oxford: Radcliffe Publishing; 2008.

Hearing the full story

9 Stern TA, Rosenbaum JF, Fava M *et al*. The optimal healing environment: patient-centered

care. *Massachusetts General Hospital Comprehensive Clinical Psychiatry*. Philadelphia, PA: Mosby; 2008.

10 Stuart M, Lieberman J, op. cit.

Authentic and active listening

11 Clabby JF. Helping depressed adolescents: a menu of cognitive-behavioral procedures for primary care. *The Primary Care Companion to the Journal of Clinical Psychiatry* 2006; **8:** 131–41.

12 Clabby J, O'Connor R. Teaching learners to use mirroring techniques to build rapport: communication lessons from neurolinguistic programming. *Family Medicine* 2004; **36:** 541–3.

Managing time

13 Marvel M, Epstein R, Flowers K *et al.* Soliciting the patient's agenda: have we improved? *Journal of the American Medical Association* 1999; **281:** 283–7.

14 Belzer E. Improving patient communication in no time. *Family Practice Management* 1999; **6:** 23–8.

15 Marvel *et al.*, op. cit.

16 Lutton M. Sticking the landing: how to create a clean end to a medical visit. *Family Practice Management* 2004; **11:** 51–3.

Cognitive therapy: Thinking creates emotions

17 Ellis A, Gordon J, Neenan M *et al. Stress Counselling: a rational emotive behaviour approach*. London: Cassell; 1997.

18 Ellis A, Harper R. *A Guide to Rational Living*. 3rd edn. Chatsworth, CA: Wilshire Book Company; 1997.

19 Jenkins D, Palmer S. Counselling in action: a multimodal assessment and rational emotive behavioural approach to stress counselling: a case study. *Counselling Psychology Quarterly* 2003; **16:** 265–87.

20 Clabby J. Helping depressed adolescents: a menu of cognitive-behavioral procedures for primary care. *The Primary Care Companion to the Journal of Clinical Psychiatry* 2006; **8:** 131–41.

Social problem solving: Helping clients to resolve their own difficulties

21 D'Zurilla T, Goldfried M. Problem solving and behavior modification. *Journal of Abnormal Psychology* 1971; **78:** 107–26.

22 Elias M, Clabby J. *Building Children's Problem-Solving and Decision-Making Skills: a school-based approach to prevention and remediation*. San Francisco, CA: Jossey-Bass; 1992.

23 D'Zurilla T, Nezu A. *Problem-Solving Therapy: a positive approach to clinical intervention*. 3rd edn. New York: Springer Publishing; 2007.

24 Malouf J, Thorsteinsson E, Schutte N. The efficacy of problem solving therapy in reducing mental and physical health problems: a meta-analysis. *Clinical Psychology Review* 2007; **27**: 46–57.

25 Cuijpers P, van Straten A, Warmerdam L. Problem solving therapies for depression: a meta-analysis. *European Psychiatry* 2007; **22**: 9–15.

26 Huibers M, Beurskens A, Bleijenberg G *et al.* The effectiveness of psychosocial interventions delivered by general practitioners. *Cochrane Database of Systematic Reviews* 2003; **2**: CD 003494.

27 Nezu A, Nezu C, Jain D. Social problem solving as a mediator of the stress–pain relationship among individuals with non-cardiac chest pain. *Health Psychology* 2008; **27**: 829–32.

28 Oxman T, Hegel M, Hull J *et al.* Problem-solving treatment and coping styles in primary care for minor depression. *Journal of Consulting and Clinical Psychology* 2008; **76**: 933–43.

Solution-focused advising: From misery talk to positive talk

29 Walter J, Pelter J. *Becoming Solution-Focused in Brief Therapy.* Levittown, PA: Brunner/Mazel, Inc.; 1992.

30 Hanton P. Solution-focused therapy in a problem-focused world. *Healthcare Counselling and Psychotherapy Journal* 2009; **9**: 22–5.

31 Berg I, Miller S. *Working with the Problem Drinker: a solution-focused approach.* New York: Howarth; 1992.

32 Corcoran J, Pillai V. A review of the research on solution-focused therapy. *British Journal of Social Work* 2009; **39**: 234–42.

33 Hanton P, op. cit.

34 Corcoran J, Pillai V, op. cit.

35 Corcoran J, Pillai V, op. cit.

36 Lipsey M. Design sensitivity: statistical power in applied experimental research. In: Bickman L, Rog D, eds. *Handbook of Applied Social Research Methods.* Thousand Oaks, CA: Sage Publications; 1998.

37 Corcoran J, Pillai V, op. cit.

38 Walter J, Pelter J, op. cit.

39 Walter J, Pelter J, op. cit.

40 Walter J, Pelter J, op. cit.

Motivational advising: Actions speak louder than words

41 Levensky E, Forcehimes M, O'Donohue W *et al.* Motivational interviewing: an evidence-based approach to counseling helps patients follow treatment recommendations. *American Journal of Nursing* 2007; **107**: 50–8.

42 Miller W, Rollnick S. Ten things that motivational interviewing is not. *Behavioural and Cognitive Psychotherapy* 2009; **37**: 129–40.

43 Thornbury S. *How to Teach Grammar.* Edinburgh: Pearson Longman; 1999.

44 Hettema J, Steele J, Miller W. Motivational interviewing. *Annual Review of Clinical Psychology* 2005; **1**: 91–111.

45 Rubak S, Sandboek A, Lauritzen T *et al.* Motivational interviewing: a systematic review and meta-analysis. *British Journal of General Practice* 2005; **55**: 305–12.

46 Miller W, Rose G. Toward a theory of motivational interviewing. *American Psychologist* 2009; **64**: 527–37.

47 Botelho R. *Beyond Advice: becoming a motivational practitioner*. Rochester, NY: Motivate Healthy Habits; 2002.

48 Ibid.

48 Prochaska J, DiClemente C. Stages and processes of self-change of smoking: toward an integrative model of change. *Journal of Consulting and Clinical Psychology* 1983; **51**: 390–5.

50 Miller W, Rollnick S. *Motivational Interviewing: preparing people to change addictive behavior*. New York: Guilford Press; 1991.

51 Deci E, Ryan R. An adaptation from self-determination theory: what motivates people to change? In: Skinner H, ed. *Promoting Health Through Organizational Change*. San Francisco, CA: Benjamin Cummings; 2002. pp. 113–14.

Eating, sleeping, smoking, and drinking

DEVELOPING HEALTHY EATING HABITS: SELF-ESTEEM, ASSESSMENT, AND TRACKING

Although the popular media and scientific literature focus much attention on obesity, policy efforts to address this problem have been rare compared with those designed to address other behavioral health risks, such as smoking. Obesity, more than smoking or problem drinking, contributes to chronic medical conditions, lower quality of life, and increased healthcare spending.[1-3] In North America, nearly one-third of the population is obese, and according to the World Health Organization obesity has become a global epidemic, actually affecting more people than hunger.[4] Based upon Wang and Beydoun's meta-analysis,[5] 66% of U.S. adults were overweight or obese, 16% of children and adolescents were overweight, and 34% were at risk of becoming overweight in 2003–2004. The fastest increase in the rate of obesity and being overweight was observed in women aged 20–34 years. Around 80% of black women aged 40 years old or older are overweight, and 50% are obese. Less educated people have a higher prevalence of obesity, with the exception of black women, according to the study. It is estimated that if the rate continues to increase like this, by 2015 75% of adults and nearly 24% of American children will be overweight or obese.

Obesity is costly. Research published in 2009[6] graphically illustrates the alarming economic costs of obesity. The annual medical burden of obesity has risen to almost 10% of all medical spending. Across all payers, the per capita medical costs for the obese are $1,429 higher per year, or nearly 42% higher, than for individuals of normal weight.[6] And diminished worker productivity is estimated at half the total cost burden.[7] Because so many clients struggle with what could become the number one preventable cause of death in the U.S., advisors needs to be familiar with some practical strategies.

The U.S. Department of Health and Human Services report sets the tone by presenting the basics.[8] Weight gain relates to the imbalance between calories consumed and calories used. And while genetics certainly play a role, much of what accounts for the recent increase in the prevalence of obesity in the U.S. is a result of changes in people's diets and level of physical activity. Clients need to attend to both aspects of the energy balance equation. Regarding energy expenditure, there is an increasingly clear and understandable consensus.[9] For example, the American Academy of Sports Medicine and the United States Department of Agriculture recommend at least 30 minutes of moderate physical activity four times weekly. Unfortunately, similarly clear and followable guidelines do not seem to exist for the energy intake side of the equation. The advisor's role is to make as clear as possible several specific behavioral changes that fit with a particular client's lifestyle. This is an effort to implement the old English proverb, "Don't dig your grave with your own knife and fork."

Assessing calorie intake can be challenging for clients to understand and for advisors to effectively communicate. However, these considerations can be broken down and made simpler. For example, the advisor can recommend that the client becomes skilled at purchasing healthy foods in the supermarket. This starts with knowing how to look for some of the particularly important facts on food labels. The most important skill is to know the serving size and how many of these serving sizes the package contains. If the client is going to eat two or three servings, they need to multiply the key nutritional facts, such as quantity of carbohydrates, by two or three, respectively.

Fiber plays an important role in weight management for two key reasons. It helps to curb the urge to eat because the body feels full, and it helps to maintain intestinal regularity. The advisor should recommend that the client purchases products that have a minimum of three or more grams of fiber per serving.

The client should look at the total amount of fat, which should be three grams or less for every 100 calories. Sugar should be kept within reasonable bounds as well. The total amount of sugar in grams is already calculated into the total carbohydrate number. The number of grams of sugar listed should be no more than one-third of the total amount of carbohydrates.

The rule of three is one way to remember the key food label facts. There should be three grams of fiber per serving, three grams of fat per 100 calories, and one-third or less grams of sugar in the total carbohydrates.

The client should only purchase products that contain mostly monounsaturated or polyunsaturated fat, and should avoid foods that tend to contain saturated fat. Foods that contain trans fats should be avoided altogether.

Advising that focuses on performing such mathematical calculations of food content may miss the mark with some clients. An advisory approach that focuses more on motivation and practical eating habits can be more effective in these cases. Some authors[10] have made weight management recommendations that are easier to follow, and their work has helped to shape some of the following suggestions.

Assuming that any medical concerns influencing weight gain have been ruled out by a physician, for some people maintaining a healthy weight may be helped on the energy intake side of the equation by knowing more about which foods are healthy and in what quantities. An advisor can refer clients to a certified nutritionist, who is a health professional with four years of undergraduate education in nutrition and often a Master's degree in nutrition as well. Clients can also read one of the many books on nutrition which present the facts about calories, carbohydrates, poly- and monosaturated fats, sugars, and their interaction. However, the most skilled advisors and nutritionists will focus on making the necessary eating behavior changes understandable and easy to follow. Informing overweight clients that they can reduce the risk of developing some chronic medical conditions by losing as little as 5–15% of their body weight[11] is a great motivational start for those clients who tend to overwhelm themselves with unrealistic expectations.

Daily records of weight and consumption

The advisor can choose to keep things simple by focusing on the effect of the greater availability of pre-packaged foods, the relatively inexpensive and large-portioned restaurant meals, and the soft drinks that are high in sugar, calories, and/or fat. Physicians most often counsel their patients along these topic lines. However, such conversations rarely include attention to two of the most well-known predictors of weight loss, namely self-weighing and recording daily intake.[12,13] The advisor should encourage clients to weigh themselves daily and to become experts on their own daily consumption. The client should record exactly what is consumed and at what times, including breakfast, lunch, dinner, and snack times such as coffee breaks. For most people, this simple intervention creates a healthy pre-occupation with sensible eating. The client can keep a food diary to monitor food intake, the events that trigger eating, and at what times. The recording of timing can yield such information as whether the client eats much of the day's calories at night, which can lead to sleep problems. There are a number of excellent practical self-recording tools available.[14]

Breakfast helps with weight management

Around 20–30% of adults in the U.S. skip breakfast.[15] This is a lost opportunity because, after adjusting for confounding variables, people who do not eat breakfast have a significantly higher body mass index than those who eat bread or cereal for breakfast.[16] Clients who do not eat breakfast, for example skip this meal 75% of the time, have a 4.5-fold increased odds of being obese compared with those who eat breakfast regularly.[17] How and where the breakfast is eaten, as well as what is eaten, is relevant. It seems that avoiding a rushed breakfast is important, and the client should allow at least 20 minutes for this important meal.[18] Having breakfast at home is a major benefit. There is evidence that eating breakfast away from home can actually double the risk of obesity compared with having breakfast at home.[19] And eating either ready-to-eat or cooked cereal or quick breads for breakfast is associated with a significantly lower body mass index compared with either skipping breakfast or eating a breakfast of meat and/ or eggs.[20]

Eating at home is important

The amount of calories that people consume per eating occasion is greater for food prepared away from home than for food prepared at home.[21] People who eat restaurant or fast food have significantly higher odds of being overweight than people who do not eat fast food.[22] There is a positive relationship between how often people eat restaurant or fast food and the increase in their body weight.[23] And the trend towards eating away from home is accelerating. Between 1977 and 1996, the average person aged 2 years or older showed an increase in restaurant and fast food consumption from 9.6% to 23.5%.[24] Healthy behaviors at restaurants include ordering more baked or broiled items rather than fried foods, controlling the intake of dressings and sauces by asking the server to place them in a side cup, and watching portion sizes. In the U.S., between 1977 and 1996 the size of the food portions consumed has been increasing even for meals that are eaten at home. However, this is an especially relevant issue for fast food restaurants, which serve the largest food portions.[25] The problem is that people eat more when larger portions of food are presented to them.[26,27] They take in 30% more food and energy when a server presents them with a 1000-g portion of food as compared with a 500-g portion. A 1000-g portion is a typical restaurant portion.[28]

Drinking beverages without sugar

Drinking beverages that contain added sugar, such as sodas, fruit drinks, and other soft beverages, has a major impact on weight gain, as these beverages account for over 40% of sugar added to the average U.S. diet.[29,30] Teenagers who increase their intake of sugar-added beverages increase their total energy intake, and they gain weight as a result. It is particularly important to address the intake of fruit juices and sweetened iced teas, because these are perceived as natural, and many well-meaning parents are not aware of the effect on weight gain of the sugar content of such beverages. Over a 1-year period, boys who drank one or two sugar-added beverages a day significantly increased their BMI by 0.10 and 0.14, respectively, and girls who consumed two or more sugar-added beverages per day significantly increased their BMI by 0.10.[31] Water, as the original beverage, is still the best beverage to recommend for managing weight.

Fruit and vegetables

The advisor should give the client an easily remembered way to identify the valued low-energy foods. Simply put, low-energy foods tend to have a high water and fiber content, as is found in fruits and vegetables, whereas high-energy foods tend to have a high content of fat.[32] Unfortunately, the increases in energy intake associated with high-energy foods do not seem to be compensated for by increased energy expenditure, thus resulting in a positive energy balance.[33] Middle-aged women who eat 1.9 servings of fruits daily have a 25% lower risk of obesity compared with women who eat fewer servings.[34] And women who eat 2.8 servings of vegetables daily have a significantly lower risk of weight gain compared with those who eat fewer servings.[35]

Eating mindfully is important

When people eat, they should focus on that activity. The electronic entertainment industry is designed to capture people's attention, and is skilled at doing so. When an individual is preoccupied with another activity (e.g. surfing the Internet, watching TV or speaking on the phone), they lose awareness of how much and what kinds of food they are eating. The advisor should ask the client to be wary of eating while otherwise occupied. Clients who eat with greater awareness, and who slowly savor their food, not only better manage their consumption but will also experience greater pleasure. A small behavior change like putting the fork or spoon down between bites slows down consumption and allows the individual to actually appreciate the pleasure of eating delicious food. Eating mindfully also means avoiding using food to satisfy needs other than hunger. This means that people should avoid eating food to calm down when they are angry, to provide comfort when they are lonely, or to provide energy when they are tired or thirsty. Sometimes these feelings can appear to be feelings of hunger. The advisor can teach the client a self-assessment tool, derived from the substance abuse treatment field, that will help them when they feel a strong urge to use food. It is called *HALT: Do I feel Hungry? Angry? Lonely? Tired or Thirsty?* Identifying these emotions helps the client to appropriately use other solutions, rather than eating food, such as mindful breathing to minimize anger, calling a friend when feeling lonely, taking a nap when feeling tired, and drinking water when feeling thirsty.

Ordering restaurant food properly is a significant health-promoting skill. Clients who are successful in managing restaurant food tend to know what they will order before they arrive at the restaurant. They may avoid unhealthy temptations by not examining the menu too much. Instead, such clients will control portion size by ordering an appetizer only, or even by ordering the children's portion. Such clients know as they leave home and on their way to the restaurant that they will only order items that are baked, broiled, grilled, or poached, and they will avoid items that are fried, crispy, breaded, or creamy.

Enjoying desserts that are healthy, such as fruits, non-fat frozen yogurt and sherbets, is important. At the same time, the advisor can encourage the client to check the caloric content of the non-fat desserts, since the sugars that are added could raise the caloric content significantly. The client should try to avoid eating commercially baked products, as these often have hidden sources of saturated fats.

Protein, such as the lean proteins of fish, chicken, turkey, loin or round cuts of beef/pork, beans, soy, nuts, or eggs, is an important component of a healthy diet. This is because protein is more filling than carbohydrates. Generally speaking, white meat is preferable to red meat. Red meat has more total fat than the white meat of chicken and turkey. And if the client wants to make an even more sophisticated weight-conscious choice, they can choose the white meat of turkey, because it is leaner than its chicken counterpart. Fish, especially shellfish, is better than either red or white meat because of its low total and saturated fat content.

Supermarket behavior is relevant, too. The advisor can suggest the general guideline of shopping the perimeter of the store, as this area most often contains the healthier whole foods, such as fruits, vegetables, dairy products, and meats, rather than the interior aisles of the supermarket, which contain the more processed and less healthy foods, such as the junk food snacks which should be kept out of the home.

Having healthy foods conveniently in supply at home is a key factor. The supermarket trip should bring home such foods as frozen vegetables, whole-wheat pasta, low-fat cheese, canned tomatoes, canned beans, precooked chicken, whole-grain pita breads/tortillas, and bagged salad. Having such easily prepared foods available at home will minimize the temptation to pick up fast food on the way home from work, or to have pizza delivered.

The Idaho Plate Method is a helpful and simple guide to healthy choices and portions. In this procedure, the advisor suggests that the client should ensure that 50% of the plate is occupied by vegetables, 25% by lean protein, and 25% by whole grains.[36] A side plate could have a low-fat dairy product or fruit for dessert.

Exercising the leg muscles is smart. During physical exercise the muscles consume fat and sugar. Because of the relatively large size of the leg muscles compared with the muscles of the rest of the body, exercising these particular muscles by walking, running, and cycling is the most efficient exercise for reducing fat.[37] Even during moderate exercise such as a brisk walk, the body shifts toward greater use of fat as a fuel.[38,39] For those clients who may be unenthused about walking for exercise, the advisor can recommend a pedometer. Using such a tool seems to fuel some motivation. In a review of 26 studies, people who used pedometers increased their level of physical activity by 26.9% over their baseline.[40] Another excellent motivator is exercising with other people. Children, for example, report that their friends help them to initiate physical activity, and modeling and co-participation by a peer who is already engaged in the activity is helpful.[41] Although exercise as it is practiced in the general population has only modest effects on weight loss, a dose–response curve exists because very intense workouts lead to substantial weight loss. During 5 months of basic military training and no dietary restriction, obese soldier recruits lost on average 12.5 kg (27.6 lb).[42]

The Cochrane Collaboration published a meta-analysis of 43 randomized trials and reported that exercising alone results in limited weight loss. However, the action of combining exercise with healthy dietary change led to a 1 kg weight loss compared with dieting alone. A 1.5 kg (3.3 lb) weight loss was observed with higher levels of exercising.[43]

Having positive self-regard while being overweight

For many clients, information is necessary but insufficient for actual habit change to take place. Many obese people have known since childhood that regularly eating super-sized hamburgers at fast food restaurants causes weight gain. Yet they continue to eat that way. For them, knowledge or the light is necessary but insufficient to cause change. In habit change, motivation is referred to as the heat. It is about the drive towards a comfortable warm heat or the drive to escape a burning heat. For many obese adults, change is not about the light, but about the heat. If a person has reasonable knowledge about sensible nutrition facts, and many obese people do, the advisor needs to avoid repeating the facts that are already known. Rather, they need to identify and cultivate the client's motivation to change, and attend more to the heat than the light. The following is one example of how to do this.

The advisor should begin by laying the motivational foundation of honoring and loving one's body as it is now. It does no good for overweight clients to dislike or hate their bodies. This self-critical attitude destroys their motivation to lose weight. Overweight clients need to accept, respect, and even love their bodies as they currently appear.[44] This is a radical idea, but one that is necessary for nutritional health. Choosing self-acceptance and a positive self-regard, despite being overweight, increase the client's motivation to change.

The advisor can tell the following story.

Advisor: "Imagine, if you wish, that you had for a long time wanted to buy a top-of-the-line suit to wear on special occasions. This suit was great-looking. It was the perfect weight, the right cut, an outstanding color, great fabric, and therefore quite expensive. If you were wearing this suit you would probably avoid playing ball in it.

You would be concerned that the suit might become soiled or torn. You would be careful about volunteering to cook at the picnic, because you would want to avoid spilling food on your expensive and great-looking suit. While wearing your suit, you would avoid working in the garden or painting your home. When changing out of your suit at the end of the day, you would probably handle it with care, perhaps hanging it on a special hanger in the closet."

Client: "Yes, I think so."

Advisor: "Now imagine that you found an old, color-faded, and rather worn suit in the back of your closet. If you wore this older suit, how would you be treating it? You wouldn't hesitate as much about wearing the suit while playing ball outside. It would be OK to get dirt on it, and even a tear in the fabic would be tolerable.

After all, it's a beat-up old suit anyway that no one cares about. It is so old, worn out, and frayed that you would be OK wearing it while you touched up a wall with paint or worked in the garden or cooked out-of-doors. In fact, when you change out of this old suit you might even just drop it on the floor in a heap. You feel no need to hang this suit up carefully. It is such a mess that it is not worth the trouble.

Actually, because you hate this suit so much, you have planned on cutting it up to use as cleaning rags for your dirty car. You really do not care about this suit and you act accordingly. You

> hate this old suit's appearance and you just would not take care
> of it properly, so it gets worse and worse looking. This old worn
> suit does not get the same respect that you would give to that
> expensive suit."

Clients need to honor their bodies, admire them, and love them now, in the same way that they would honor that expensive and attractive new suit. This is the message that the advisor can impart to the client who is concerned about being overweight or out of shape. Some religious traditions actually regard the body as a spiritual temple. If clients respect their bodies as they are right now, regardless of their shape or appearance, they will be more likely to treat their bodies well with proper exercise, sleep, and nutrition.

Understanding the medicines for weight management allows the advisor to make a significant contribution in preparing the client for discussions with their physician about both the prescription and over-the-counter (OTC) medicines. There are clients who have medical, not cosmetic, reasons for losing weight, who have been doing all the right things, such as exercising regularly and eating properly, but who are still not losing weight. These clients would benefit from asking a physician about the benefits of adding weight-loss medicines.

Prescription drugs have been approved by the Food and Drug Administration (FDA) for those clients who have a body mass index (BMI) of 30 or above, or who have a BMI of 27 plus an obesity-related condition such as hypertension, type 2 diabetes, or dyslipidemia (abnormal amounts of fat in the blood). These FDA-approved drugs for weight loss are appetite suppressants in that they give an individual the feeling of being full by increasing one or more of the brain chemicals that affect appetite. The two most commonly prescribed appetite suppressants in the U.S. are sibutramine and phentermine. Sibutramine is approved for use for up to one year in adults. One of the common side-effects listed is increased blood pressure and heart rate. Phentermine has been approved for use for up to 12 weeks in adults. In addition to the possible side-effect of higher blood pressure and increased heart rate, it can also cause sleeplessness and nervousness. Diethylpropion is also approved for short-term use (up to 12 weeks) in adults, and its possible side-effects include dizziness, headache, sleeplessness, and nervousness. In addition, phendimetrazine is approved for use for up to 12 weeks in adults, and its possible side-effects include sleeplessness and nervousness.

Another FDA-approved anti-obesity drug is orlistat (Xenical), which is not an appetite suppressant but a lipase inhibitor. Lipase is the enzyme responsible for breaking down dietary fat. When the medicine inhibits lipase from breaking down the fat, the body cannot absorb the fat so it is eliminated, and fewer calories are taken in. This drug has been FDA approved for use for up to one year in adults, and its common side-effects include gastrointestinal problems such as cramping, diarrhea, and oily spotting.

In 2007, orlistat was approved for OTC sale to adults aged 18 years or older. Now a prescription is no longer needed and it is marketed as Alli. It is intended to be used in conjunction with a reduced-calorie, low-fat diet, regular exercise, and a daily multi-vitamin. The side-effects of Alli are similar to those of the prescription form of orlistat. Clients who are considering taking Alli should be educated about the side-effects listed above, drug interactions, and the usage recommendations.[45]

Advisors can also provide clients with information resources to support healthy eating. The American Dietetics Association, which is the professional organization for registered dieticians, has a helpful website (www.eatright.org). The United States Department of Agriculture (USDA) also has a useful website (www.My Pyramid.gov). These sites provide motivational suggestions, an interactive online supportive community, customized meal planners based upon a client's personal goal, recipes, meal-planning worksheets, and food consumption tracking sheets. Clients can even obtain feedback on how much progress they are making in their efforts. There are other free support organizations, such as Overeaters Anonymous, as well as for-profit organizations such as Weight Watchers.

To help to maintain the client's motivation, the advisor should be aware of the findings of the National Weight Control Registry (NWCR), the purpose of which is to identify the common characteristics of over 4800 individuals who have succeeded in maintaining their weight loss.[46] There may be a common misconception that few people succeed in the long term in keeping the weight off. However, the evidence indicates that approximately 20% of overweight individuals succeed in achieving long-term weight loss, defined as loss of at least 10% of the initial body weight, and that they maintain that loss for at least one year. It is further reported that members of the NWCR have lost an average of 33 kg and maintained the weight loss for more than 5 years. Moreover, maintaining weight loss may become easier over time, since after keeping the weight off for two to five years, the likelihood of even longer-term success greatly increases.[47]

There are some common behaviors that these people used to maintain the weight loss. They utilized a combination of healthy eating and daily exercise. No specific diet was followed, but rather these individuals focused on low calories and low fat content, and chose foods with a higher carbohydrate content. They also exercised for an hour each day, with walking being the most popular choice of activity. They would eat four to five times per day, and breakfast was an important part of their daily routine, as was watching only a limited amount of television. While some clients might regard this as boring, the people who lost and kept off the weight limited their dining out to no more than three times per week, and they consistently ate the same kinds of meals, including on weekends and holidays. They wrote down daily what they ate, and they weighed themselves often. If they noticed a small weight gain, they took quick action to readjust their lifestyle.[48,49]

POSITIVE STEPS FOR A GOOD NIGHT'S SLEEP

Insomnia is difficulty in initiating or maintaining sleep, or not having the type of sleep that is refreshing and restorative. It causes significant stress and impaired work and social functioning. Approximately one-third of adults report symptoms of insomnia, 9–12% experience additional daytime consequences, and approximately 6% meet the formal criteria for a diagnosis of insomnia.[50,51] Clients with insomnia often simply report that they are not getting enough rest or sleep despite their best efforts, and that they feel dissatisfied or frustrated by this. These clients cite such symptoms as taking 30 minutes or longer to fall asleep, or they report that once they are finally asleep they wake up and then struggle to get back to sleep, or they describe waking up too early in the morning, and well before the alarm. These clients report that as a result they experience difficulty with memory, a lower threshold for irritability and anger, absenteeism from work, interpersonal conflicts with co-workers, family, and friends, tiredness and low energy, and impaired automobile driving that can contribute to injuries or death.

There are two major types of insomnia. The first is *transient insomnia* which is a common response to environmental and situational stressors. With this type, cognitive–behavioral therapy (CBT) strategies, such as sleep hygiene, can be quite helpful. This section focuses on these kinds of strategies. A second type of insomnia, which is termed *persistent insomnia*, can be a red flag for a number of possible physical diseases and conditions, including menstrual pain, medication side-effects, frequent urination at night, serious psychiatric problems, substance abuse, menopause, and sleep apnea (which involves a narrowing of the upper airway during sleep, with night-time symptoms such as snoring, snorting, and gagging). In cases of persistent insomnia, it is important that the advisor recommends that the client should see a physician who can gather a complete history and perform a physical examination to identify the underlying cause. As appropriate, a physical medicine solution can be safely offered along with the CBT strategies discussed in this section.

Sleep disorders are expensive, and are associated with an estimated cost of $15 billion per year in the U.S.[52] Data was submitted in 2007 and published in 2009 that estimated the total annual cost of insomnia in the province of Quebec alone at $6.6 billion Canadian dollars. This includes the costs of insomnia-related medical consultations ($191.2 million), transportation for these consultations ($36.6 million), prescription medications ($16.5 million), OTC products ($1.8 million), and alcohol used as a sleep aid ($339.8 million). Annual indirect costs associated with insomnia-related absenteeism were estimated at $970.6 million, with insomnia-related productivity losses estimated at $5.0 billion.[53]

Some insomnia is caused by behavioral habits that are not conducive to getting restful sleep, and many healthcare providers are unaware of the usefulness and effectiveness of ways to treat insomnia without using medications.[54] A review of the collective findings of four well-controlled randomized studies suggests that CBT produces significantly greater subjective and objective sleep improvements compared with no treatment, pharmacologic interventions, non-pharmacologic placebo interventions, and progressive muscular relaxation training. These same four studies also indicate that the sleep improvements which result from CBT tend to endure across a range of post-treatment follow-up periods, ranging from 3 to 24 months.[55] One study reports that combined CBT and pharmacotherapy (temazepam) may produce slightly greater short-term sleep benefits than CBT alone.[56] The results of that study indicate that people who received CBT alone showed better maintenance of their improved sleep than did those who received the combined CBT and pharmacotherapy. In summary, a variety of behavioral treatments have been shown to be effective in empirical studies and also offer many advantages over medications, including in many cases being more effective in the long term than medication.[57] A menu of CBT strategies from which the advisor and client can choose is described below.

Sleep hygiene education

In addition to using behavioral approaches, the client can also see a physician who can determine whether prescription sleeping medications would help them to fall asleep more easily, stay asleep longer, or both. By the time the client talks to an advisor, they may have tried some of the OTC sleep aids, including antihistamine-based products, such as Nytol, and other sleep aid supplements, including melatonin, valerian, hops, and chamomile. None of these are regulated by the U.S. Food and Drug Administration (FDA). Although some randomized, controlled trials have been conducted for a few compounds, rigorous scientific data supporting a beneficial effect have not been obtained for the majority of herbal supplements, dietary changes, and other nutritional supplements that are widely used to treat insomnia symptoms.[58]

Caffeine stimulates the central nervous system. Because it provides a temporary energy boost and increases alertness, sleep-deprived clients may use caffeine for this purpose in the daytime. Caffeine is found in tea, coffee, chocolate, and many soft drinks. Some clients may not be aware of the amount of caffeine that they are consuming, because it is also found in pain relievers and other OTC medications. It is understandable why a sleep-deprived client would use caffeine to stay alert during the day, but this creates a problem later when the client wants to sleep. A recent review of the evidence concludes that caffeine abstinence for a whole day can improve the quality of sleep, and it therefore recommends that advisors include caffeine abstinence as an instruction in sleep hygiene advice for clients with insomnia.[59]

The advisor should recommend that the client keeps a sleep journal to record what triggers the restless sleep. For example, they should note the activities engaged in just before bedtime, the time when the client actually gets into bed, the number of occasions and the exact time when the client wakes up during the night, the total number of hours slept, what (if anything) disturbed the sleep, and the time when the client gets up in the morning. Using such information, the advisor can discuss the impact on sleep of diet, especially foods eaten 2 or 3 hours before bedtime, possible alcohol use, the timing and duration of physical exercise, and specific environmental factors such as light, noise, and temperature. Good sleep hygiene also involves the client trying to schedule potentially agitating conversations, physical exercise, substantial meals, and electronic media entertainment for much earlier in the day. They should wind down their activities several hours before bedtime, and start spending time the way people did generations ago before electricity extended the day (e.g. by enjoying a physically sedating warm bath, reading a calming book, and so on).

Sleep restriction is a very helpful technique for a client who wants to overcome insomnia. It involves limiting the amount of time during which the client is restlessly tossing and turning in bed. The client should be in bed only for the average amount of time of actual sleep. For example, they may have to get out of bed for work by 07.00 am, and they may be averaging 6½ hours of sleep per night. With sleep restriction, the client should go to bed no earlier than 12.30 am, because the initial recommended sleeping window would be restricted to 6½ hours. Adjustments to this initial recommended window can gradually be made as the client slowly begins to average more sleep (e.g. 6¾ hours, 7 hours, and so on).

Stimulus control

The client should organize their bedtime routine and rituals so that they become automatic. For example, they would walk the dog at the same time, lock the doors for the night when they return home from the walk, then bathe, brush their teeth, change for bed, and ensure that they are in bed at the same time each evening. Even if the night before was not particularly restful, the client should always go to bed and get up at the same time. Sleeping in at the weekend and napping to make up for lost sleep must stop. The client should get up each day at the same time regardless of the length and quality of the previous night's sleep. A cool room temperature, a comfortable pillow, and keeping the room dark are three important factors that promote good sleep. When the client is trying to drift off to sleep, their body should not have to work to stay warm or cool. The advisor should recommend that the client only goes to bed when they feel sleepy. If sleep has not come within 15 or 20 minutes, they should get out of bed and go and sit on a nearby comfortable chair or sofa and read a boring book or article. In the cooler months, the client should keep a blanket or robe nearby to use while they are sitting in the chair or on the sofa. Once they have begun to feel sleepy again, the client can return to bed. They should get up at the same time every morning, and eliminate naps.

A major feature of stimulus control is regarding the bedroom as a relaxing refuge. Too often the bedroom has become a second office – a place where people handle weekend and evening work calls, write and receive reports, send text messages, faxes, and email, and even work on trying to balance budgets. The bedroom then becomes associated with the pressured feelings of solving problems and meeting deadlines. It is difficult to turn this industrious energy off and relax when the client can still see the digital clock, computer, and other electronic communication devices that ignite a recall of the never-ending to-do list. The bedroom has also become an additional electronic entertainment center. Rather than unwinding, people become energized and agitated while engaging in competitive video or computer games or rooting for a favorite sports team on a wide-screen TV. When using stimulus control to eliminate insomnia, the bedroom should be a relaxing, pleasant, peaceful environment that is associated only with the pleasures of sleep and sex. Some of the strategies that are described later in the stress management chapter can be quite helpful. Again, consultation with a physician is very important for managing physical medical problems such as sleep apnea.

SMOKING CESSATION

Helping those who are not yet ready to quit

Tobacco use accounts for 435,000 deaths every year in the U.S., where it is regarded as the major avoidable cause of illness and death.[60] Therefore developing advisory approaches to help tobacco users to quit is literally a matter of life and death.[61] Despite the increased research on smoking, heightened awareness of its consequences, and considerable publicity about litigation against tobacco companies, the Centers for Disease Control and Prevention (CDC) has reported that an estimated 44.5 million adults in the U.S. smoke cigarettes, and more than 8.6 million of them have at least one serious illness caused by smoking.[62] In the 18–24 years age group, smoking rates actually increased by 32% between 1991 and 1997.[63]

Despite their unfortunate use of tobacco, clients who smoke also want to live long and healthy lives. In fact, 70% of physicians' patients who smoke say that they would like to quit.[64] The challenge confronting smokers who want to quit is formidable. This is graphically illustrated by, for example, patients with smoke-induced throat cancer who continue to smoke through the tracheotomies in their necks,[65] and starving refugees who trade their food rations for cigarettes. Although 70% of patients who smoke say that they would like to quit, only 7.9% are able to do so without help.[66] However, there is hope, because we now know that something relatively low cost, such as the advice of an advisor (e.g. a physician) alone, can increase the smoking cessation rate to 10.2%.[67] The question then is what forms of advice yield the best outcomes.

Most smokers know that smoking is harmful. Teachers, relatives, friends, and healthcare providers have been preaching about this or admonishing clients about the habit for years. Clients who smoke have also seen plenty of anti-smoking slogans on highway billboards and in other print media. They have heard messages on the radio and television about the harmful effects of nicotine. Many have experienced social ostracism, such as being told that they cannot smoke at a worksite, being forbidden to smoke in restaurants, or have felt embarrassed by the implication that they are being irresponsible.

Providing facts is necessary but insufficient to facilitate such change. The piling on of alarming medical predictions is an approach that has failed many clients who smoke. Furthermore, such techniques create an adversarial relationship between the advisor and the client. Motivational interviewing avoids such tactics. It maintains that quitting smoking is not so much about medical knowledge. After all, there are many people, such as physicians, who have a high level of medical knowledge and still smoke. Change is about the client's vivid emotional excitement about the fact that quitting will contribute to many positive factors. Change also relates to believing that quitting is achievable. Clients smoke because they are physically addicted, because they like the stress reduction experience that they believe smoking provides, or because they greatly value what they see as its weight-reducing benefits. The advisor's focus should be on the client's emotions and helping them to believe that they can access the tools which will work to enable them to quit.

When the topic of smoking cessation comes up, it is efficient to pause and recognize the person's readiness to change.[68] This builds rapport, guides the choice of questions that the advisor will ask, and minimizes the likelihood of the unintended outcome whereby the client is even more convinced to smoke. A respectful and helpful way to begin the conversation would be for the advisor to ask "What are your thoughts and feelings about quitting?"

In the motivational interviewing approach, the pre-contemplators are simply not ready to quit. A client could come across as defiant (e.g. "I like to smoke and that's that"), ignorant of the facts (e.g. "I already smoke a low-tar cigarette, so there's no need to quit"), angry (e.g. "Look, that's not what I came to talk to you about, OK?"), entitled (e.g. "Look, I'm a nurse, I think I know the situation"), or in denial (e.g. "Some people get lung cancer from smoking, but that doesn't happen in my family"). The advisor should avoid pushing back, because this just intensifies the person's resistance to quitting. The role of the advisor is to respectfully and gently plant doubt in the client's belief that they cannot change. This can be done in at least four ways, as described below.

The first approach is to use past failure as an asset. The National Cancer Institute's Cancer Information Service of the U.S. National Institute of Health reports that people commonly quit smoking only to find themselves taking up the habit again. This is particularly likely to occur in the first few weeks or months after quitting. When clients are discouraged about this, the advisor should explain that most people who smoke after quitting should try to quit again. In fact, it may take four or more attempts before smokers are able to quit for good.[69] Here is an example of a dialogue using this approach.

Advisor: "Have you tried to quit before?"

Client: "Yes. It didn't work out."

Advisor: "I'm sorry about that. It's strange, but that actually might be quite helpful. (Pause) Usually a number of quit efforts are needed before it works. It's like a new skill that needs to be learned" *or*

"That's actually OK. People who have tried to quit before tend to use those experiences because it helps them plan more successful quitting strategies" *or*

"It's interesting, quitting is actually a learning process that gets stronger over time."

The second approach is to build on the client's past successes. Many clients have taken on such difficult challenges as moving to a new city or country, succeeding in a difficult job, successfully raising a family, or managing and balancing a budget during difficult economic times. And many of them take for granted the success that they have had in handling such complex challenges. The advisor can authentically and respectfully reflect on this aloud: "When you are ready to stop smoking, my sense is that you will be successful, like you were with the other hard things you have done in your life, such as working two jobs to support your family."

The third approach is to elicit the client's projections. The advisor finds out about the client's worries and concerns, and then uses this information to intensify the client's motivation to quit. The advisor could say "Many people have quit smoking. Why do you imagine all those people have quit?" The client may answer "Maybe they're worried about the cost." No matter what the client says, the advisor should acknowledge the ideas and/or agree. Whatever the response, it is probably a projection of the client's own concerns, as they will have little idea why other people quit. Then the advisor can help to deepen this projected motivation by asking "How much does a pack of cigarettes cost these days?"

The fourth approach is to raise positive expectations. The advisor uses the word "when" as opposed to the word "if", as this implies the inevitability that the client will quit. For example, the advisor could remark "You know that wheezing in your chest will get a lot better when you quit smoking." They avoid saying "if you quit" but, instead say "when you quit" or "after you quit." The observations should be individualized, specific, and positively predictive of smoking cessation.

Clients who are at the next stage of change are actually considering quitting and are described as contemplators. They are intrigued but remain ambivalent, and are not quite ready to make the move. Such clients might say "Maybe I will stop. Yeah, I'm thinking about quitting." Here the advisor helps the client to commit to the healthy change that they want. The advisor should anchor quitting to what the client is really excited about achieving in life. They should facilitate the client to do most of the talking, because it is the client's personal thoughts and feelings that are central. The motivational interviewing approach unfolds in the following step-wise fashion:

1 The advisor and client **agree to an agenda**, with the advisor stating "Great. So it sounds like you want to decide whether to stop smoking or not."

2 **The advisor asks about the advantages of smoking** and then summarizes: "I know you must be sensing some advantages of smoking. Tell me about those." It is easier for a client to let go of a behavior if they honestly acknowledge the value of that bad habit. When an advisor asks about this value, the client often finds this a relief. It is often experienced as a positive, therapeutic surprise to be able to share thoughts and feelings about the benefits of smoking. The advisor would summarize by stating. For example, "So, an advantage of smoking is that it gives you a rare moment in your busy day to be alone and relax."

3 **The advisor next asks about the disadvantages of smoking**, and summarizes that understanding as well. For example, "At the same time, you are sensing some disadvantages of smoking. Tell me about those." This is still respectful, because the agenda from the beginning was to have an open discussion about whether to quit smoking or to continue. The advisor would then summarize. For example, "The disadvantages you see are that smoking lowers your physical stamina and it costs more and more money each year."

4 Next, **the advisor asks about the client's hopes and plans** and then summarizes: "If things worked out in the best possible way for you, what are you looking forward to and excited about doing in a year?" The focus is on facilitating the client's expression of these positive and exciting goals. A client's vision of a desired, happy, and satisfying future is the energy source that powers the motivation to change. Once the advisor has heard the client's hopes and plans, they summarize: "So if things worked out well for you in one year, you would be running in the park with your grandson, buying him little treats like ice cream, going swimming, and having the healthiest heart and blood pressure you could possibly have. That's great!"

   Unfortunately, the more typical approach to advising pits the advisor and the client against each other. The advisor would strongly advocate or argue for change while the client would politely and quietly sit and listen, or self-righteously resort to defending their decision to smoke. This old approach backfires, with the client becoming even more entrenched in the bad habit. In the motivational interviewing approach, the advisor and client join forces as a team to fight the obstacles that are in the way of the client's hopes and plans.

5 **The advisor then develops a healthy discrepancy and asks for a decision.** With a caring, quizzical look they would slowly say "I'm not sure how smoking helps you get there." The advisor would then remain silent for a moment. This can feel like an awkward moment, but it is a therapeutic one. The advisor should avoid rescuing the client from this awkwardness and let the discrepancy sink in a little. This often provides the tipping point for the client to decide to make the healthy change. The advisor can state "When we started our talk your goal was to decide whether to stop smoking or not. Where are you now with your decision?" The client might simply state "You know, it just doesn't make sense anymore for me to carry on smoking. I need to quit." Some clients may be quiet with their own thoughts at this point. Others, not knowing how to proceed, may start talking about something else. The advisor can help by praising the client for engaging in the discussion, and offering to discuss the matter again if the client wishes to do so.

Many clients move from the pre-contemplation stage of change to the contemplation stage of change, and then to the readiness-to-change stage. They will make comments such as: "I want to figure out a way to finally quit, and this time I have to make it permanent." The advisor's goal is now to help the client to make a plan, implement it, maintain the healthy change, and prevent relapse. This includes making such recommendations as choosing a quit date, obtaining social support by making the decision to quit publicly known to family members, co-workers, and friends, and getting rid of ash trays and other similar reminders of smoking. In addition, the advisor should encourage the client to see a physician to discuss the use of medicines that can help them, and to make contact with a support network such as a telephone quitline, both of which are discussed below.

The National Cancer Institute's Cancer Information Service of the U.S. National Institute of Health has a variety of resources available for smoking cessation, including helpful products that contain nicotine and equally helpful products that do not. Nicotine is the substance in cigarettes and other forms of tobacco that causes addiction. Nicotine replacement products provide small, measured doses of nicotine which help to relieve the cravings and withdrawal symptoms that are often experienced by clients who are trying to quit. There is strong and consistent evidence that nicotine replacement products do help clients to quit smoking.[70] Unlike tobacco smoke, these products do not contain large numbers of toxic and cancer-causing substances. The long-term use of nicotine replacement products is not known to be associated with any serious harmful effects.[71] All nicotine replacement products, which are approved by the FDA and available as a patch, gum, lozenge, nasal spray, or inhaler, appear to be equally effective. The advisor should recommend that the client consults with their physician regarding which product would best suit the client's individual circumstances and lifestyle. Under a physician's supervision, clients can discuss issues such as quitting tobacco use before using nicotine replacement products,[72] as too much nicotine can cause nausea, vomiting, dizziness, weakness, diarrhea, or rapid heartbeat. For some clients, physicians might advise combining the nicotine patch with nicotine gum or nicotine nasal spray, as for them this may work better than using a single type of nicotine replacement therapy.[73,74] Nicotine gum combined with nicotine patch therapy may reduce withdrawal symptoms more effectively than either medication alone. The patch provides a baseline level of nicotine, and the additional products can deliver extra doses of nicotine when cravings or withdrawal symptoms occur. All of these nuances of treatment strongly support the value of consulting a physician.

Bupropion is among the products that aid smoking cessation and which do not contain nicotine. A prescription antidepressant, marketed as Zyban, it was approved by the FDA in 1997 to treat nicotine addiction. Bupropion can help to reduce nicotine withdrawal symptoms as well as the urge to smoke,[75] and can be used safely with nicotine replacement products.[76] Again, the advisor should suggest that the client arranges a consultation with a healthcare provider so that they can ask questions and decide whether this product, like the others mentioned, would be appropriate for their needs. Varenicline is another of the prescription medicines that does not contain nicotine. It is marketed as Chantix™, and was approved for smoking cessation by the FDA in 2006. This drug aims to ease withdrawal symptoms, and also to block the effects of nicotine from cigarettes if the smoker relapses. Another option is a combination of bupropion and nicotine patch therapy.[77,78] Again, the advisor should suggest that the client consults with a physician before deciding whether this treatment is appropriate for them.

The popular media and word of mouth have both influenced smokers to consider trying approaches such as hypnosis, acupuncture, laser therapy, and electro-stimulation to help to reduce the symptoms associated with withdrawal from nicotine. A client may tell the advisor about someone for whom one of these approaches worked. That person's perspective should be respected. Although it is understandable that a frustrated client may want to try one of these techniques, as yet there are no clinical studies showing that these techniques help people to quit smoking.[79] What can be recommended are specialist smokers' clinics, which provide services that are beyond what can be offered through brief consultation with a primary care physician such as a family doctor.[80]

There are many government and private non-profit organizations that support clients who are considering quitting. Among the most effective services offered are the various telephone-based programs known as quitlines. The client calls a quitline, where the services can include mailed materials, recorded messages, counseling at the time of the call, callbacks from the counselor, access to nicotine cessation medicine, or various combinations of these services. Most of these services are cost-free. Quitline assistance is available in the U.S. in all 50 states and in Washington, DC, through a single national telephone portal (1-800-QUIT NOW). This is sponsored by the National Network of Tobacco Cessation Quitlines, an initiative of the Department of Health and Human Services (HHS), and it routes the client to a state-run quitline that provides the help. National quitlines are available in Europe and many Asian countries, as well as in a few South American countries.[81] Quitlines have many advantages.[82] First, phone counseling eliminates many of the logistical barriers to accessing services. If the client needs more time and help, they can just call the quitline back and resume where they left off. Second, quitlines can be time efficient, because the semi-anonymous nature of the phone conversation makes many clients feel comfortable and able to be candid. This allows the quitline counselor to obtain an accurate picture of the situation quite quickly. Third, the telephone allows the counseling to be proactive in that the quitline counselor can initiate calling the client back. This increases the likelihood that follow-ups will take place. This proactive counseling encourages accountability by providing social support. Fourth, the telephone format allows for a structured counseling format which provides some minimal acceptable and focused content.

The evidence in support of the effectiveness of quitlines is strong,[83] and is based upon randomized controlled trials of large samples that include diverse populations. For example, two large trials in California each included more than 3,000 smokers, a high proportion of ethnic minority smokers, and were conducted in both English and Spanish.[84,85]

The advisor can also recommend the following resources.

➤ The Tobacco Control Research Branch of the National Cancer Institute (NCI), a component of the National Institutes of Health, established the Smokefree.gov website in collaboration with the Centers for Disease Control and Prevention and the American Cancer Society to help people to quit smoking. The website (www.smokefree.gov) provides information in English and Spanish.

➤ The National Cancer Institute (NCI) Smoking Quitline offers individualized counseling in English or Spanish, Monday through Friday,

9.00 a.m. to 4.30 p.m. (local time), printed information, referrals to other sources, and recorded messages. Tel: 1-877-448-7848 (1-877-44U-QUIT); website: www.cancer.gov

➤ The National Institute on Drug Abuse (NIDA) offers information on drug abuse and addiction in English and Spanish. NIDA publications can be ordered from the National Clearinghouse for Alcohol and Drug Information (NCADI). Tel: 1-800-729-6686 (1-800-SAY-NO-TO), 240-221-4019, 1-877-767-8432 (for Spanish-speaking callers); website: http://ncadi.samhsa.gov

➤ The Agency for Healthcare Research and Quality (AHRQ) issues smoking cessation guidelines and other materials for physicians, healthcare professionals, and the general public. Printed copies are available by contacting the AHRQ. Tel: 1-800-358-9295 (toll-free), 703-437-2078 (for international callers); website: www.ahrq.gov

Nonprofit organizations that can be recommended by the advisor include the following.

➤ The American Cancer Society (ACS) provides materials on quitting smoking and other smoking- and tobacco-related topics. For a local ACS office, contact the ACS's National Home Office. Tel: 1-800-227-2345 (1-800-ACS-2345); website: www.cancer.org

➤ The American Heart Association (AHA) provides information on local and community-related intervention programs in schools, workplaces, and healthcare sites, and offers brochures on quitting and the relationship between smoking and heart disease. For the telephone number of a local AHA chapter, contact AHA's national office. Tel: 1-800-242-8721 or 1-800-AHA-USA; website: www.americanheart.org

➤ The American Lung Association (ALA) provides information about local quit smoking programs as well as its Freedom From Smoking® clinics for individuals and organizations. Tel: 1-800-586-4872 (1-800-LUNG-USA) and 212–315–8700; website: www.lungusa.org

➤ Nicotine Anonymous provides group support and uses the Twelve Step approach from Alcoholics Anonymous. The website provides a searchable database of meetings by state and country. Internet and telephone meetings are also offered. Publications are available in nine languages (English, Danish, Farsi, French, German, Hungarian, Portuguese, Spanish, and Swedish). The client can contact this organization for further information. Tel: 415-750-0328; website: www.nicotine-anonymous.org

ALCOHOL USE

Prevalence and screening

According to the CDC, 64% of Americans drink alcohol, of whom 50% report that they are regular drinkers. With this level of alcohol consumption in the U.S., there were 22,073 alcohol-caused deaths in the year 2006. These are deaths that are unrelated to accidents, suicides or homicides. Half of these reported deaths are from liver disease resulting from alcohol use. Preliminary data for 2009 show the highest percentage of adults who have consumed more than five drinks a day (23%) in a decade. This may reflect the economic downturn of the significant economic recession and the related psychosocial problems related to that, including job and home loss and the various accompanying family stresses.[86] Men drink more alcohol than women, and the highest level of overall use occurs in the 18–24 years age group. Alcohol abuse rates are higher among non-Hispanic whites (27%) than among Hispanics (19%) or blacks (15%).[87]

Alcohol abuse is diagnosed if, over a 12-month period, a client shows at least one of the following recurrent behaviors: failure to fulfill major role responsibilities at work or at school due to alcohol use (e.g. repeated absences or poor performance); use of alcohol in situations where it would be physically dangerous (e.g. when driving); legal problems (e.g. arrests for disorderly behavior or driving while intoxicated); and problems with relationships (e.g. arguments and fights) that are connected to alcohol use.[88] The *Diagnostic and Statistical Manual of Mental Disorders, Fourth Edition (DSM-IV)* describes alcohol abusers as those who drink despite recurrent social, interpersonal, and legal problems occurring as a result of alcohol use.

Alcohol dependence is the diagnosis for a client whose drinking has led to significant problems as indicated by at least three of the following:

➤ tolerance, characterized by either a need for increasing amounts of alcohol in order to obtain the desired effect, or experiencing a significantly lessened effect with continued drinking of the same amount of alcohol

➤ physical withdrawal symptoms from the alcohol, or the need to use a substance to relieve or avoid those withdrawal symptoms

➤ the client drinking larger amounts of alcohol or drinking over a longer period than planned

➤ a recurrent desire or unsuccessful efforts to reduce or control the use of alcohol

➤ the client spending much time working to obtain and drink the alcohol or to recover from its impact

➤ reduced involvement in important social, recreational, or occupational activities, because of the alcohol use

➤ the client continuing to drink despite realizing that there is a persistent problem caused by the drinking.[89]

The prevalence of lifetime and 12-month alcohol abuse is reported to be 17.8% and 4.7%, respectively, and the prevalence of lifetime and 12-month alcohol dependence is reported to be 12.5% and 3.8%, respectively. Alcohol dependence has been shown to be significantly more prevalent among men, whites, Native Americans, younger and unmarried adults, and people with lower incomes. Current alcohol abuse (within the previous 12 months) was more prevalent among men, whites, and younger and unmarried individuals, while lifetime rates were highest among middle-aged Americans.[90] Alcohol abuse and dependence are associated with automobile accidents,[91] domestic violence,[92] fetal alcohol syndrome,[93] neuropsychological impairment,[94] poor medication adherence,[95] economic costs and reduced productivity,[96] and psychiatric comorbidity.[97]

Because of the high prevalence of alcohol abuse and dependence, it is a likely advising issue. With alcohol problems in particular, the advisor needs to be available and approachable, and to create an atmosphere of safety. It is not easy for a client to talk about this issue, since alcohol problems continue to be highly stigmatized, even more so than mental illnesses.[98] The client could be the person actually abusing the alcohol, but they might well also be the concerned friend, family member, or co-worker. This is because the social impact on family and friends can be among the most significant factors in leading a person to seek help. One way in which these social consequences have been expressed is through a method known as an intervention. This is a professionally guided, organized, and caring confrontation by one or more concerned individuals simultaneously.[99,100] The advisor could well be speaking with a client whose family has just completed an intervention.

Although alcohol problems are so prevalent, it is disappointing how relatively few healthcare professionals, such as primary care physicians, regularly screen their patients for alcohol problems. Only 55–65% of physicians routinely ask patients about alcohol use during the initial visit, and only 35% actually screen patients during their annual visit to the doctor.[101–103] One of the first tasks for the advisor is to ascertain the extent of the possible alcohol problem. A positive response to screening tools such as those listed below should raise the suspicion level, and prompt the advisor to investigate further and/or refer the person to a health professional who specializes in this area.

➤ **Quantity:** A standard drink is one 12-ounce bottle of beer, one 5-ounce glass of wine, or 1.5 ounces of distilled spirits. According to the National Institute on Alcohol Abuse and Alcoholism (NIAAA),[104] men may be at risk for alcohol use problems if they drink more than 14 standard drinks per week, or more than four drinks per day. For women, the equivalent figures would be more than seven standard drinks per week, or more than three drinks per day.

➤ **The 1-3-5 Question:** An advisor can gain a high yield by asking the 1-3-5 question: "On any single occasion during the past three months, have you had more than five drinks containing alcohol?" A positive response to this single question accurately identifies people who meet either the criteria for alcohol abuse or dependence, as outlined in the *Diagnostic and Statistical Manual of Mental Disorders, Fourth Edition*[105] or the NIAAA standard for at-risk drinking.[106]

➤ **Relationships, Work, and the Police:** A client may not be willing or able to report the quantity of alcohol consumed. The advisor should avoid aggressively pursuing this line of questioning, as it might alienate the client. If the amount of drinking is not revealed, or even if the quantity consumed seems to be within reasonable limits, the use of alcohol can still have a serious impact on quality of life. The advisor would simply ask "Has your drinking alcohol led to any difficulties:

— at work (e.g. being suspended, being fired, loss of promotion, lack of raises, etc.)

— in relationships (e.g. break-up of a romantic relationship, being excluded from social events with family or friends, having arguments or fights, etc.) *or*

— with the police (e.g. being arrested for driving while intoxicated, physical violence, road rage, etc.)?"

A positive response to any of these screening questions should prompt the advisor to investigate further and/or refer the client on.

➤ **The CAGE screen (Cut down, Annoyed, Guilt, Eye-Opener):** This screening tool is used internationally,[107,108] with each letter representing a standard question. Two or more positive responses are considered to be indicative of probable alcoholism, while one positive response suggests that the person's alcohol use merits further evaluation.[109] The CAGE screen is short, easy to use, and has shown high reliability as well as correlating with other screening instruments. It is not an appropriate screen for the less severe forms of drinking, and has not performed well with college students, white women and prenatal women.[110] The following is an example of its use.

Cut down:

Dr. Jackson: "Mike, have you ever tried to cut down on your drinking?"

Mike: "Once in a while."

Annoyed:

Dr. Jackson: "Do you get annoyed when people ask about your drinking?"

Mike: "Yeah, but especially when other people ask me, like my son's basketball coach of all people!"

Guilt:

Dr. Jackson: "That sounds uncomfortable. Mike, do you ever feel guilty about your drinking?"

Mike: "No, not really."

Eye opener:

Dr. Jackson: "Do you ever drink early in the morning to get your day started? Some people call it an eye opener."

Mike: "Yeah, well, I've been known to do that from time to time." (smiles)

If there is a positive response to any of these screening tools and a need for treatment, the question then becomes what treatment to recommend. As well as encouraging primary care doctors to screen adult patients for alcohol problems using brief assessment procedures,[111] the NIAA recommends that when there is a positive screen and a need for treatment, clients should be directed to either *abstinence* if they seem to be alcohol dependent or alcoholic, or *moderation* if they are not alcohol dependent.[112] In concert with these recommendations, the following is a description of these two treatment approaches.

Helping alcohol-dependent and problem drinkers to abstain

A client who is physically addicted to alcohol and wants to stop drinking completely needs to see a physician for medical treatment to stop drinking safely. When a client who has used alcohol heavily for a long time stops drinking, they may experience a range of physical symptoms that are proportional to the level of alcohol intake and the duration of the client's recent drinking pattern. The possible symptoms range from the moderate, such as insomnia, anxiety, and shaking, to the severe, such as delirium tremens (DTs). The latter is a violent delirium that includes a fading in and out of consciousness, increased motor activity, visual hallucinations, disorientation, confusion, and fever. Such a state is a medical emergency because it could be fatal.[113] Clients can undergo alcohol withdrawal in a hospital setting, and many can withdraw safely and effectively under the care of a physician as an outpatient. The physician can also then assess other complicating medical conditions (e.g. congestive heart failure, liver disease and infections, and pancreatitis), prescribe the appropriate medicine, and monitor the client throughout the detoxification experience.[114] Once a client has safely withdrawn from alcohol, they can stay under the care of a physician if ongoing medication is recommended, and/or they can enter a comprehensive rehabilitation program, which can include individual, family, and group psychotherapy as well as involvement with the 12 step program of Alcoholics Anonymous (AA), which is discussed below.

Clients with alcohol problems as well as their family members and friends who are clients can continue to help themselves before, during, and after the detoxification or rehabilitation experience and learn more about alcohol by participating in 12 step programs such as Al-Anon and AA. An advisor who is familiar with such 12 step programs will more competently and confidently assist the client to get the help that they need. A family member or friend may approach the advisor with a question such as "I'm not the person with the drinking problem. It's my husband, and it's more than I can take. I need some help." Often these family members and friends become so preoccupied with their worries about the problem drinker that they begin to neglect their own physical and psychological well-being. They find themselves caught up with such behaviors as counting how many drinks the person has had, or actually purchasing the alcohol to keep the peace, or lying to bosses to cover for the person who is drinking. Some of these clients become addicted to helping. While remaining involved in a supportive capacity, the advisor can extend the help that is available by encouraging clients to also connect with Al-Anon, the 12 step program specifically designed to support friends and family members.

The benefits of AA for the drinker who needs to abstain are often hard fought but extremely worthwhile. The advisor who understands the AA experience plays an important role in reassuring the client who is hesitant about getting started with AA. The explanation of AA described here is based on that of Kaskutas.[115] It takes significant staying power for a client to accept a referral for AA, attend a meeting and then continue to attend for the long-term benefits.[116] In fact, AA reports that 50% of the alcoholics who come to AA stop attending within the first three months.[117] The Institute of Medicine estimates that only 20% of alcoholics who are referred to AA ever attend meetings regularly.[118] AA-naive clients may feel anxious about their initial AA meeting, imagining that they will be pressured to talk about their problems or to commit to a program that they are only just learning about. Attending meetings requires effort, and might often, as Valliant[119] describes it, involve sitting on hard chairs in church basements for several times a week. The advisor can remind clients that it is the people of AA who make it more than worthwhile. As part of their own recovery, AA members commit to help others by volunteering, for example, to be a supportive, available sponsor for a new member. This involves being just a phone call or personal meeting away, to help the member who is confused about the recovery process or who needs support when they are tempted to have a drink. Other volunteer activities that aid in ongoing recovery could include preparing the coffee for the meeting, or maintaining the literature which is distributed to new members. The advisor can empathize and reassure the client that the only goal for a first AA meeting is for the client to receive information about AA. There is no pressure for a commitment. AA is indeed anonymous. The only self-identifier that participants share is a first name. At the initial meeting, the client can merely state a first name and say that they are there just to listen and learn. AA works because the meetings create a safe, encouraging atmosphere for people to share and listen to others talking about what helps them to abstain. The benefits accumulate if the client who decides to stay with AA begins to share with the group particular struggles and feelings that they are experiencing. The client learns that it is possible to live without alcohol and have reasonable expectations of him- or herself by changing one day at a time.

The steps of AA, the common curriculum, routinely remind the AA participants that alcohol has outmatched them. The AA members are asked to depend upon a higher power. This higher power might be spiritual, or it could simply be AA itself. So in the references to God in the 12 steps, the non-religiously affiliated member can substitute the concept of AA. The other steps involve accepting how one's actions have affected others, a resolve to relate to others in an improved way, committing to discovering meaning in life, and giving up on a negative focus on oneself by assisting other people.

The following are the original Twelve Steps as published by Alcoholics Anonymous.[120]

➤ Step One: We admitted we were powerless over alcohol – that our lives had become unmanageable.

➤ Step Two: We came to believe that a Power greater than ourselves could restore us to sanity.

➤ Step Three: We made a decision to turn our will and our lives over to the care of God as we understood Him.

➤ Step Four: We made a searching and fearless moral inventory of ourselves.

➤ Step Five: We admitted to God, to ourselves, and to another human being the exact nature of our wrongs.

➤ Step Six: We were entirely ready to have God remove all these defects of character.

➤ Step Seven: We humbly asked Him to remove our shortcomings.

➤ Step Eight: We made a list of all persons we had harmed, and became willing to make amends to them all.

➤ Step Nine: We made direct amends to such people wherever possible, except when to do so would injure them or others.

➤ Step Ten: We continued to take personal inventory and when we were wrong promptly admitted it.

➤ Step Eleven: We sought through prayer and meditation to improve our conscious contact with God as we understood Him, praying only for knowledge of His will for us and the power to carry that out.

➤ Step Twelve: Having had a spiritual awakening as the result of these steps, we tried to carry this message to alcoholics, and to practice these principles in all our affairs.

Kaskutas[121] discusses the theory underpinning the activities of AA, citing Bandura's social learning theory.[122] Understanding how AA works involves understanding the roles played by social influences and self-efficacy. If surrounded by people who drink and who doubt the client's ability to abstain from drinking, the chances are that the client will not be able to abstain. There are then three key solutions:

1 altering the environmental pattern, such as the client avoiding scenes where drinking is prominent (e.g. the bar, tavern, and unfortunately even some family gatherings)

2 spending time with positive role models, such as frequently going to gatherings like AA meetings where other people work hard at abstaining

3 setting reasonable expectations for oneself. Rather than self-imposing the formidable goal of quitting forever, the client would move towards not drinking, one day at a time.

Successfully abstaining for one day at a time builds up confidence. Confidence also comes from the encouragement that a client receives at AA when abstinence anniversaries and accomplishments are celebrated at the meeting. At AA, members have access to a hidden curriculum of behavioral techniques that are shared formally and informally, such as learning assertive ways of saying no to a drink when it is offered, having a plan available when faced with pressure to drink, and anticipating likely drinking conditions.

Kaskutas[123] cites a number of studies that explain some of the reasons why AA is successful. These include such psychological and spiritual mechanisms as finding meaning in life,[124] getting greater motivation for abstinence,[125] experiencing changes in the religious and spiritual domains,[126] having regular exposure to positive social influences and reducing the amount of pro-drinking influences,[127] having more friends in general,[128] having AA friends who are supportive of abstinence,[129] developing enhanced friendship networks,[130] cultivating a positive sense of self-efficacy,[131,132] and learning effective coping and relapse prevention skills, such as calling a sponsor for support when the urge to drink is particularly powerful.[133,134] These benefits work together to form a supportive fabric. Developing more friendships with people who are abstinent, being with them at AA meetings, and spending time with them in other non-drinking social venues provides access to the hidden curriculum mentioned earlier.

Helping a problem drinker who is not an alcoholic to cut down

An Institute of Medicine report found that for every one alcoholic, there are approximately three problem drinkers who are at risk for serious health problems, but who do not meet the criteria for the clinical diagnosis of alcoholism, also called alcohol dependence.[135] These problem drinkers may drink often and excessively, and may even take dangerous risks like drinking and driving. However, they have not reached the nearly total and consistent loss of control over drinking, and the series of negative consequences related to it, that characterize alcoholism. A classic problem drinker is the college student who sometimes engages in binge drinking, or the homemaker whose nightly glass of wine has turned into a nightly bottle.

The field of alcohol treatment has its share of controversies, the most significant one in the U.S. concerning Moderation Management (MM), the only mutual-help organization that offers people help in learning how to control their drinking.[136] The goal of this is to attract problem drinkers who want to change, who are not dependent on alcohol, and who are uninterested in and unmotivated by the abstinence-only approach.[137] In reaction, prominent figures in the alcohol treatment and research communities denounced MM as a dangerous temptation to alcoholics that was built on the illusion that alcoholics could return to controlled drinking.[138] This debate intensified when MM's founder, Audrey Kishline, left MM, joined AA, and several months later caused the deaths of two people in a horrific car accident while severely intoxicated.[139]

The focus on total, life-long abstinence dominates the alcohol treatment field. At the same time, there have been many theoretical, scientific, and practical arguments in favor of supplementing abstinence-oriented interventions with moderation management or controlled drinking (CD) approaches. The term "controlled drinking" is preferable, and will be used from here onward, because the other terms such as "moderation management", "normal drinking", "social drinking", "non-problem drinking", "asymptomatic drinking", and "moderate drinking", may wrongly suggest that it is an easy option compared with total abstinence. This is an unhelpful message, as controlled drinking takes a lot of work, and the client still needs to deal with the social and environmental prompts (e.g. being in a nice restaurant and having a glass of wine with animated friends with lively music playing in the background, and so on).[140]

The advisor should remember that there is compelling scientific evidence[141] that controlled drinking treatment is effective compared with alternative interventions or no treatment in decreasing both the amount and frequency of alcohol intake. It is difficult to facilitate clients at any level of alcohol consumption to get the help that they need, because of the denial, stigma, and other barriers to care. Some clients who are not physically addicted to alcohol might finally be ready to change if they understand and get solidly behind the controlled drinking strategy. There are strong beliefs about the important role played by the controlled drinking option, with some scientists stating that "we see no need to be apologetic or defensive about the CD goal, since evidence and rationality are overwhelmingly on its side."[142] Indeed, offering information and advice about the moderation option to non-dependent but problem drinkers may convince some problem drinkers to start working on behavior change. Clients will benefit if they can frankly discuss their intention to try to drink moderately, rather than hiding this intent out of shame. Providing reasonable options to the non-physically dependent drinker who declines abstinence is important, as clients are much more committed to change when they are working on self-selected goals.[143] And from an ethical stance alone, it could be argued that clients have the right to be fully informed about the pros and cons of all the available options, including abstinence and controlled drinking.

The controlled drinking approach maintains that these problem drinkers can stop or moderate when they wish. The organizing belief is that moderation is a realistic, achievable, and clinically responsible goal for many problem drinkers. It is not for everyone. For some drinkers, responsible drinking means no drinking. Controlled drinking is not meant to tempt anyone back into drinking who has found in abstinence secure resolution of a previous severe alcohol problem. Anyone who is physically dependent should be cautioned against attempting moderation, because the chances of success decline with the severity of the alcohol problem.

The advisor should recommend the following general guidelines for controlled drinking:

1 not drinking for more than three or four days per week
2 for women, an upper limit of three drinks per occasion, and not more than nine per week
3 for men, an upper limit of four per occasion, and not more than 14 per week
4 alcohol should be consumed at a slow pace
5 there should be absolutely no drinking and driving.

The advisor's message to the problem drinker who is considering controlled drinking

The message to such a problem drinker should include being clear about the problems that overdrinking has caused, and thinking positively to keep in mind the benefits of moderation, including having new activities and interests. The advisor should share the variety of techniques for dealing with the urge to drink, and for controlling drinking when the client chooses to drink. The client can then select the techniques that seem most appropriate. The client should also identify what triggers the overdrinking, and develop strategies to manage these triggers more effectively. It should be clear to the client that successful controlled drinking requires them to be hyper-focused in any drinking situation, and it is often helpful to keep a journal of what happens. The advisor should suggest that the client uses any lapses as valuable learning experiences and refuses to let them decrease motivation.

Skills for managing drinking

1 **Abstaining for the first 30 days.** The client begins the modified drinking approach by first abstaining for 30 days. Early in the process, this period of abstinence breaks old habits. It helps the client to regroup and become more sensitive to the physical and psychological sensations that can alert them that a tipping point is nearing when another drink might lead to problems.

2 **Countering irrational urges to drink more.** When a client senses that the tipping point is near (e.g. they start to have a feeling of relaxation, mild euphoria, increased gregariousness, being humorous, etc.), that is a sign that the blood alcohol level is rising and getting close to a sensible limit for moderate drinking. It is at this moment that the client may experience an irrational urge to abandon the moderate drinking strategies. This urge may come in the form of such faulty thinking as "I haven't had a break all week and I deserve a moment to relax" or "I think I can handle another drink without a problem", or "If

you can't have a few drinks at your own brother's wedding, when can you?" In this situation, the alcohol is interfering with higher-order and logical thinking. It is not easy but the client needs to recognize that these are irrational thoughts, walk away from the alcohol, stop the self-delusional thinking, and with a clear "no-nonsense" attitude stop drinking.

3   **Anticipating.** The advisor can ask the client to identify and anticipate difficult situations (e.g. a brother's lively and joyous wedding reception, when the client may be especially tempted to drink irresponsibly). Once such situations have been identified and anticipated, the advisor should ask clients to vividly imagine a movie of how they will successfully handle themselves there. The advisor can also suggest some of the techniques listed in this chapter.[144]

4   **Knowing each drink's alcohol content.** The advisor can explain what a standard drink actually is (12 ounces of regular beer, 5 ounces of wine, or 1.5 ounces of 80 proof hard liquor), and how much alcohol is in each drink. The beer is easy to track. However, wine servings can be tricky to estimate because the sizes of wine glasses vary so widely. The advisor can suggest that the client practices by pouring 5 ounces of water into a glass at home to get a good idea of what this amount really looks like. The same thing holds for hard liquor. A person needs to become skilled at knowing ahead of time what 1.5 ounces really looks like. Measuring the alcohol content of mixed drinks such as punches or martinis is difficult, so it may be best to avoid mixed drinks altogether in such circumstances.

5   **Keeping an Alcohol Report Card.** The advisor should explain to the client that at any moment the client should be able to answer the question "How many drinks have I had so far today?" Away from the view of others, some clients have written this down for themselves. This healthy vigilance helps to prevent over-eating, and it also works for controlled drinking.

6   **Guarding the first 5 minutes.** The advisor should also recommend that the client resists the impulse to rush to the bar in order to start drinking. Clients should take time to get a feel for the social situation, and perhaps start with a non-alcoholic beverage. When having a first alcoholic drink, the client should mindfully savor the taste and sip it slowly. The first 5 minutes often set the pace for the rest of the event, and the client should delay the onset of drinking and slow the pace down from the start.

7   **Drinking water.** Responsible drinkers hydrate themselves with water or a non-alcoholic drink before even going to a gathering where alcohol will be served. The urge for a beer, for example, could actually be an urge to quench a thirst. Many clients who are successful at drinking moderately satisfy their thirst in a responsible manner well before the event.

8 **Arriving late and leaving early.** Those who are skilled at controlled drinking recognize their vulnerability and are kind to themselves by limiting their exposure to alcohol. They tend to deliberately arrive late at the event. Once there, they delay the time at which they have their first alcoholic drink. They also tend to leave the event before the others do.

9 **Eating food is good.** Eating before drinking or while drinking slows down the time it takes for the alcohol to get into the system and exert its effects. The client is then less likely to be taken unawares by the effects of the alcohol, which makes it easier to recall and implement these moderation strategies.

10 **Diluting the alcohol.** Drinks with a lower concentration of alcohol take longer to be absorbed into the body. Even a hard liquor drink on ice alone can be diluted by adding a mixer such as tonic water. A glass of wine can be converted into a lighter alcoholic drink by mixing it with a seltzer to make a wine cooler. The client could also handle the social pressure from others to drink excessively by continually re-filling their drink with a mixer.

11 **Switching to something special.** Some clients avoid drinking alcoholic beverages in succession. They order or mix themselves a sophisticated-looking non-alcoholic alternative such as an orange-cranberry drink with seltzer over ice in an attractive glass. They then switch to such a non-alcoholic beverage in between consuming alcoholic drinks. The client can take the time to sip, savor, and appreciate the non-alcoholic drink, which also reduces their anxiety about not having something to hold.

12 **Savoring a beverage.** Some clients allow themselves to consume alcohol after a very demanding work or family day when they have had to move quickly under pressure to get everything done. They make the mistake of continuing at the same frenetic pace when they encounter alcohol, by tossing beers down, and so on. The advisor can help the client to become aware of this tendency, by suggesting that they just slow down and savor the full experience of what they are doing. It is a deadly race to feel compelled to catch up with others or to have to hustle to be next to get the bartender's attention.

13 **Finding a table.** This technique is incredibly simple and effective. The advisor recommends that whether the client is sitting or standing, they should always put the glass or bottle down on a table. This obliges the client to have to make a small effort to reach for the beverage. This encourages more conscious choices about the number of sips that are taken. It minimizes the more mindless reflex action of the elbow automatically bending to bring a drink to the mouth. A client who may feel awkward if they do not have something to hold in their hand can plan ahead and have something else

to hold, such as a swizzle stick, napkin, business card, or even a car key.

14 **Clocking it.** Clients benefit by determining ahead of time how many drinks they can safely handle on a particular occasion. They then can decide at what time it would be safe for them to begin the drink. For example, a client might think "I can have up to two alcoholic drinks tonight. If I want to have a second drink, I will wait at least one hour between drinks."

15 **Taking alcohol seriously.** Successful clients think about, plan, and take their personal and work relationships seriously. This avoids problems. The same is true about alcohol. To give this challenge of alcohol the dignity that it deserves, clients who learn controlled drinking take a moment and ask themselves "Do I want this beer because I am thirsty? If so, maybe I'll have a glass of water first", or "Am I calm enough to savor this beer and not rush?", or "Will this drink get in the way of what I have planned for the rest of the evening, such as being able to drive home or keeping a promise to my partner?"

16 **Shopping first.** The advisor can suggest that clients avoid being dependent on what the hosts of the party will be serving. Instead, they can take control by shopping for themselves. They can keep a variety of their own favorite healthy beverages available at home and bring these to social gatherings.

17 **Remembering priorities.** The manufacturers of alcoholic beverages would want clients to think it is all about the beer. However, that kind of message is a problem. Clients should remind themselves that the gathering can be less about the alcohol and more about the playing or the viewing of the game with friends, or laughing or having good conversations. The companionship of friends can be deliberately savored. The client can make it more about the friends and football, and less about the alcohol.

18 **Being sharp for tomorrow morning.** The advisor can encourage the client to literally think ahead about what they would like to have happen the next morning. For the parents of young children, it may be to enjoy a Saturday of playing with them without the irritability that accompanies a hangover. For a student, it may be about being focused enough to finish a research paper and meet a deadline. For a client who is concerned about looking attractive, it may be about feeling physically well enough to go to the next day's workout at the gym in order to continue losing weight.

19 **Having a back-up plan.** The advisor can suggest that the client should expect the unexpected. For example, part of a client's controlled drinking plan may be to avoid a bar during the working week. They could anticipate that an important professional contact might spontaneously suggest a meeting at the hotel bar to discuss a lucrative deal. The client could graciously accept

the offer to meet, and enthusiastically suggest a meal at a nice restaurant instead. Some clients say that they are watching their health and fitness and need to be careful about what they are eating and drinking. Others, when needing some encouragement to stay strong, pull out a photograph of a family member or friend who would be so pleased if the controlled drinking continued. Other clients, in the 12 step tradition, might call a sober support person and talk things over.

20 **Using drink refusal skills.** The advisor can prepare clients to be respectfully assertive in a clear and firm manner when others exert pressure on them to drink. The client can adjust their Posture, Language, Use of eyes, and Sound of voice (PLUS)[145] to present a clear message.

— Posture relates to standing or sitting in a steady and still businesslike stance.

— Language refers to such options as saying no, changing the subject (e.g. "Never mind that drink, Bob, hey, I wanted to ask you, how is work these days?"), suggesting an alternative activity such as getting something to eat or having a non-alcoholic drink (e.g. "No, not for me, Bob, but those chips look good"), simply being direct and avoiding offering a rationale or explanation (e.g. "You know Bob, I said I don't want a drink. No need to ask me again. Thanks"). Some people persist in putting on the pressure. In such cases the client should simply avoid offering explanations, as these just provide material that the persistent person will use to counter-argue. The client can just simply repeat the same brief message (e.g. "Bob, as I said, no drink for me. No need to ask me again"). If the person persists and is just not getting the message, it may be that they are intoxicated, in which case the client can just walk away.

— Use of eyes directs the client to have a non-threatening but direct and steady gaze.

— Sound or tone of voice often trumps the language. So even if the client does not choose the best words, it is more the firmness, strength, and no-nonsense quality of the voice tone that wins out.

— As one final note, clients perform better in terms of assertiveness if they practice it by role playing with the advisor first. If PLUS can be overlearned through practice, it will be easier to use when it is really needed in an anxious, pressured moment.

Putting things into context, it is important to remember that even the alcohol consumption of the majority of normal drinkers is occasionally risky or even harmful in relatively minor ways. Depending on the person who is drinking and the situation, there is no level of drinking that is entirely risk-free.[146]

REFERENCES

Developing healthy eating habits: Self-esteem, assessment, and tracking

1 Long A, Reed R, Lehman G. The cost of lifestyle health risks: obesity. *Journal of Occupational and Environmental Medicine* 2006; **48**: 244–51.

2 Sturm R. The effects of obesity, smoking, and drinking on medical problems and costs: obesity outranks both smoking and drinking in its deleterious effects on health and health costs. *Health Affairs (Millwood)* 2002; **21**: 245–53.

3 Finkelstein E, Fiebelkom I, Wang G. National medical spending attributable to overweight and obesity: how much, and who's paying? *Health Affairs (Millwood)* 2003; **Jan-Jun, Suppl. Web Exclusives (W3):** 219–26.

4 Powers K, Jones S. Financial impact of obesity and bariatric surgery. *Medical Clinics of North America* 2007; **91**: 321–38.

5 Wang Y, Beydoun M. The obesity epidemic in the United States – gender, age, socioeconomic, racial/ethnic, and geographic characteristics: a systematic review and meta-regression analysis. *Epidemiologic Reviews* 2007; **29**: 6–28.

6 Finkelstein E, Trogdon J, Dietz W. Annual medical spending attributable to obesity: payer- and service-specific estimates. *Health Affairs (Millwood)* 2009; **28**: 822–31.

7 US Department of Health and Human Services. *Prevention Makes Common "Cents": executive summary.* Washington, DC: US Department of Health and Human Services; 2003.

8 Ibid.

9 Greenwood J, Stanford J. Preventing or improving obesity by addressing specific eating patterns. *Journal of the American Board of Family Medicine* 2008; **21**: 135–40.

10 Ibid.

11 US Department of Health and Human Services, op. cit.

12 Phelan S, Nallari M, Darroch F *et al.* What do physicians recommend to their overweight and obese patients? *Journal of the American Board of Family Medicine* 2009; **22**: 115–22.

13 Wing R, Tate D, Gorin A *et al.* A self-regulation program for maintenance of weight loss. *New England Journal of Medicine* 2006; **355**: 1563–71.

14 Hark L, Deen D. Taking a nutrition history: a practical approach for family physicians. *American Family Physician* 1999; **59**: 1521–8.

15 Cho S, Dietrich M, Brown C *et al.* The effect of breakfast type on total daily energy intake and body mass index: results from the Third National Health and Nutrition Examination Survey (NHANES III). *Journal of the American College of Nutrition* 2003; **22**: 296–302.

16 Ma Y, Bertone E, Stanek E *et al.* Association between eating patterns and obesity in a free-living US adult population. *American Journal of Epidemiology* 2003; **158**: 85–92.

17 Ibid.

18 Ortega R, Redondo R, Lopez-Sobolar A *et al.* Associations between obesity, breakfast-time

food habits and intake of energy and nutrients in a group of elderly Madrid residents. *Journal of the American College of Nutrition* 1996; **15**: 65–72.

19 Ma Y, Bertone E, Stanek E *et al.*, op. cit.

20 Cho S, Dietrich M, Brown C *et al.*, op. cit.

21 Nielsen S, Siega-Riz A, Popkin B. Trends in energy intake in U.S. between 1977 and 1996: similar shifts seen across age groups. *Obesity Research* 2002; **10**: 370–8.

22 Bowman S, Vinyard B. Fast food consumption of U.S. adults: impact on energy and nutrient intakes and overweight status. *Journal of the American College of Nutrition* 2004; **23**: 163–8.

23 Pereira M, Kartashov A, Ebbeling C *et al.* Fast-food habits, weight gain, and insulin resistance (the CARDIA study): 15-year prospective analysis. *Lancet* 2005; **365**: 36–42.

24 Guthrie J, Hwan B, Frazao E. Role of food prepared away from home in the American diet, 1977–78 versus 1994–96: changes and consequences. *Journal of Nutrition Education and Behavior* 2002; **34**: 440–50.

25 Nielson S, Popkin B. Patterns and trends in food portion sizes, 1977–1998. *Journal of the American Medical Association* 2003; **289**: 450–3.

26 Levitsky D, Youn T. The more food young adults are served, the more they overeat. *Journal of Nutrition* 2004; **134**: 2546–9.

27 Diliberti N, Bordi P, Conklin M *et al.* Increased portion size leads to increased energy intake in a restaurant meal. *Obesity Research* 2004; **12**: 562–8.

28 Rolls B, Morris E, Roe L. Portion size of food affects energy intake in normal-weight and overweight men and women. *American Journal of Clinical Nutrition* 2002; **76**: 1207–13.

29 Guthrie J, Morton J. Food sources of added sweeteners in the diets of Americans. *Journal of the American Dietetic Association* 2000; **100**: 43–51.

30 Johnson R, Frary C. Choose beverages and foods to moderate your intake of sugars: the 2000 dietary guidelines for Americans – what's all the fuss about? *Journal of Nutrition* 2001; **131**: 2766–71S.

31 Berkey C, Rockett H, Field A *et al.* Sugar-added beverages and adolescent weight change. *Obesity Research* 2004; **12**: 778–88.

32 Rolls B, Drenwnoswski A, Ledikwe J. Changing the energy density of the diet as a strategy for weight management. *Journal of the American Dietetic Association* 2005; **105**: 98–103.

33 Stubbs R, Ritz P, Coward W *et al.* Covert manipulation of the ratio of dietary fat to carbohydrate and energy density: effect on food intake and energy balance in free-living men eating ad libitum. *American Journal of Clinical Nutrition* 1995; **62**: 330–7.

34 He K, Hu F, Colditz G *et al.* Changes in intake of fruits and vegetables in relation to risk of obesity and weight gain among middle-aged women. *International Journal of Obesity and Related Metabolic Disorders* 2004; **28**: 1569–74.

35 Rolls B, Row L, Meengs J. Salad and satiety: energy density and portion size of a first-course salad affect energy intake at lunch. *Journal of the American Dietetic Association* 2004; **104**: 1570–6.

36 Rizor HM, Richards S. "All our patients need to know about intensified diabetes management they learned in fourth grade." *The Diabetes Educator* 2000; **26**: 392–404.

37 Gwinup G. Weight loss without dietary restriction: efficacy of different forms of aerobic exercise. *American Journal of Sports Medicine* 1987; **15**: 275–9.

38 Sahlin K, S Allstedt E, Bishop D *et al.* Turning down lipid oxidation during heavy exercise –what is the mechanism? *Journal of Physiology and Pharmacology* 2008; **59(Suppl. 7)**: 19–30.

39 Haskell W, Lee I, Pate R *et al.* Physical activity and public health: updated recommendations for adults from the American College of Sports Medicine and the American Heart Association. *Circulation* 2007; **116**: 1081–93.

40 Bravata DM, Smith-Spangler C, Sundaram V *et al.* Using pedometers to increase physical activity and improve health: a systematic review. *Journal of the American Medical Association* 2007; **298**: 2296–304.

41 Jago R, Brockman R, Fox KR *et al.* Friendship groups and physical activity: qualitative findings on how physical activity is initiated and maintained among 10–11 year old children. *International Journal of Behavioral Nutrition and Physical Activity* 2009; **6**: 1–9.

42 Lee L, Kumar S, Leong LC. The impact of five-month basic military training on the body weight and body fat of 197 moderately to severely obese Singaporean males aged 17 to 19 years. *International Journal of Obesity and Related Metabolic Disorders* 1994; **18**: 105–9.

43 Shaw K, Gennat H, O'Rourke P *et al.* Exercise for overweight or obesity. *Cochrane Database of Systematic Reviews* 2006; **Issue 4**: CD003817. DOI:10.1002/14651858. CD003817. pub3.

44 Cruise J. *8 Minutes in the Morning for Real Shapes, Real Sizes: specifically designed for people who want to lose 30 pounds or more.* Ashford, UK: Rodale Books; 2005.

45 Weight-control Information Network (WIN). *Prescription Medications for the Treatment of Obesity.* WIN-07-4191. Bethesda, MD: National Institute of Diabetes and Digestive and Kidney Diseases (NIDDK), National Institutes of Health; 2004 (revised 2007).

46 Hill J, Wyatt H, Phelan S *et al.* The National Weight Control Registry: is it useful in helping deal with our obesity epidemic? *Journal of Nutrition Education and Behavior* 2005; **37**: 169.

47 Wing R, Phelan S. Long-term weight loss maintenance. *American Journal of Clinical Nutrition* 2005; **82(Suppl.)**: 222–5S.

48 Ibid.

49 Hill J, Wyatt H, Phelan S *et al.*, op. cit.

Positive steps for a good night's sleep

50 Morin C, Bootzin R, Buysse D *et al.* Psychological and behavioral treatment of insomnia: update of the recent evidence (1998–2004). *Sleep* 2006; **29**: 1398–414.

51 Ohayon M. Epidemiology of insomnia: what we know and what we still need to learn. *Sleep Medicine Reviews* 2002; **6**: 97–111.

52 Weilburg J, Richter J. The patient with disordered sleep. In: Stern T, Herman J, Slavin P, eds. *Massachusetts General Hospital Guide to Primary Care Psychiatry.* New York: McGraw-Hill Companies, Inc.; 2004. pp. 251–61.

53 Daley M, Morin D, Leblanc M *et al.* The economic burden of insomnia: direct and indirect

costs for individuals with insomnia syndrome, insomnia symptoms, and good sleepers. *Sleep* 2009; **32**: 55–64.

54 Chesson A, Anderson W, Littner M *et al.* Practice parameters for the non-pharmacologic treatment of chronic insomnia. An American Academy of Sleep Medicine report. Standards of Practice Committee of the American Academy of Sleep Medicine. *Sleep* 1999; **22**: 1134–56.

55 Edinger J, Means M. Cognitive-behavioral therapy for primary insomnia. *Clinical Psychology Review* 2005; **25**: 539–58.

56 Morin C, Colecchi C, Stone J *et al.* Behavioral and pharmacological therapies for late-life insomnia: a randomized controlled trial. *Journal of the American Medical Association* 1999; **281**: 991–9.

57 Ebben M, Spielman A. Non-pharmacological treatments for insomnia. *Journal of Behavioral Medicine* 2009; **32**: 244–54.

58 Meolie A, Rosen C, Kristo D *et al.* Oral nonprescription treatment for insomnia: an evaluation of products with limited evidence. *Journal of Clinical Sleep Medicine* 2005; **1**: 173–87.

59 Sin CW, Ho JS, Chung JW. Systematic review on the effectiveness of caffeine abstinence on the quality of sleep. *Journal of Clinical Nursing* 2009; **18**: 13–21.

Smoking cessation

60 Centers for Disease Control and Prevention. Annual smoking-attributable mortality, years of potential life lost, and productivity losses – United States, 1997–2001. *Morbidity and Mortality Weekly Report* 2005; **54**: 625–8. www.cdc.gov/mmwr/previw/mmwrhtml/mm5425a1.htm (accessed 23 November 2010).

61 Lichtenstein E, Shu-Hong S, Tedeschi G. Smoking cessation quitlines: an under-recognized intervention success story. *American Psychologist* 2010; **65**: 252–61.

62 Weinstein N, Slovic P, Waters E *et al.* Public understanding of the illnesses caused by cigarette smoking. *Nicotine and Tobacco Research* 2004; **6**: 349–55.

63 Rigotti N, Lee J, Wechsler H. US college students' use of tobacco products: results of a national survey. *Journal of the American Medical Association* 2000; **284**: 699–705.

64 Fiore M, McCarthy D, Jackson T *et al.* Integrating smoking cessation into primary care: an effectiveness study. *Preventive Medicine* 2004; **38**: 412–20.

65 Sieggreen M. The power of nicotine addiction. *Tobacco Control* 1993; **2**: 315–16.

66 Fiore M, McCarthy D, Jackson T *et al.*, op. cit.

67 Jorenby D, Fiore M. The Agency for Health Care Policy and Research smoking cessation clinical practice guideline: basics and beyond. *Primary Care* 1999; **26**: 513–28.

68 Prochaska J, DiClemente C, Norcross J. In search of how people change: applications to addictive behaviors. *American Psychologist* 1992; **47**: 1102–14.

69 Kotlyar M, Hatsukami D. Managing nicotine addiction. *Journal of Dental Education* 2002; **66**: 1061–73.

70 Stead L, Perera R, Bullen C *et al.* Nicotine replacement therapy for smoking cessation. *Cochrane Database of Systematic Reviews* 2008; **Issue 1**: CD000146. DOI: 10.1002/14651858. CD000146.pub3.

71 Molyneux A. Nicotine replacement therapy. *British Medical Journal* 2004; **328:** 454–6.

72 George T, O'Malley S. Current pharmacological treatments for nicotine dependence. *Trends in Pharmacological Science* 2004; **25:** 42–8.

73 Molyneux A, op. cit.

74 Kotlyar M, Hatsukami D, op. cit.

75 Shiffman S, Johnston J, Khayrallah M *et al.* The effect of bupropion on nicotine craving and withdrawal. *Psychopharmacology* 2000; **148:** 33–40.

76 George T, O'Malley S, op. cit.

77 Kotlyar M, Hatsukami D, op. cit.

78 Jorenby D, Leischow S, Nides M *et al.* A controlled trial of sustained-release bupropion, a nicotine patch, or both for smoking cessation. *New England Journal of Medicine* 1999; **340:** 685–91.

79 White A, Rampes H, Ernst E. Acupuncture for smoking cessation. *Cochrane Database of Systematic Reviews* 2002; **Issue 2:** CD000009.

80 West R, McNeil A, Raw M. Smoking cessation guidelines for health professionals: an update. *Thorax* 2000; **55:** 987–99.

81 Lichtenstein E, Shu-Hong S, Tedeschi G, op. cit.

82 Zhu S-H, Tedeschi G, Anderson C *et al.* Telephone counseling for smoking cessation: what's in a call? *Journal of Counseling and Development* 1996; **75:** 93–102.

83 Lichtenstein E, Shu-Hong S, Tedeschi G, op. cit.

84 Zhu S-H, Anderson C, Tedeschi G *et al.* Evidence of real-world effectiveness of a telephone quitline for smokers. *New England Journal of Medicine* 2002; **347:** 1087–93.

85 Zhu S, Stretch V, Balabanis M *et al.* Telephone counselling for smoking cessation: effects of single-session and multiple-session interventions. *Journal of Consulting and Clinical Psychology* 1996; **64:** 202–11.

Alcohol use

Prevalence and screening

86 US Department of Health and Human Services, Centers for Disease Control and Prevention, National Center for Health Statistics. *Summary Health Statistics for U.S. Adults: National Health Interview Survey, 2008.* Hyattsville, MD: National Center for Health Statistics; 2009.

87 US Department of Health and Human Services, Centers for Disease Control and Prevention, National Center for Health Statistics. *Early Release of Selected Estimates Based on Data from the January–September 2009 National Health Interview Survey. Alcohol consumption.* Hyattsville, MD: National Center for Health Statistics; 2010.

88 American Psychiatric Association. *Diagnostic and Statistical Manual of Mental Disorders, Fourth Edition (DSM-IV).* Washington, DC: American Psychiatric Association; 1994.

89 Ibid.

90 Hasin D, Stinson F, Ogburn E *et al.* Prevalence, correlates, disability, and comorbidity of DSM-IV alcohol abuse and dependence in the United States: results from the National

Epidemiologic Survey on Alcohol and Related Conditions. *Archives of General Psychiatry* 2007; **64**: 830–42.

91 Chou S, Dawson D, Stinson F *et al*. The prevalence of drinking and driving in the United States, 2001–2002: results from the National Epidemiologic Survey on Alcohol and Related Conditions. *Drug and Alcohol Dependence* 2006; **83**: 137–46.

92 Caetano R, Nelson S, Cunradi C. Intimate partner violence, dependence symptoms and social consequences from drinking among white, black, and Hispanic couples in the United States. *American Journal on Addictions* 2001; **10(Suppl.)**: 60–69.

93 Lemoine P, Harousseau H, Borteyru J *et al*. Children of alcoholic parents – observed anomalies: discussion of 127 cases. *Therapeutic Drug Monitoring* 2003; **25**: 132–6.

94 Bates M, Bowden S, Barry D. Neurocognitive impairment associated with alcohol use disorders: implications for treatment. *Experimental and Clinical Psychopharmacology* 2002; **10**: 193–212.

95 Tucker J, Burnam M, Sherbourne C *et al*. Substance use and mental health correlates of nonadherence to antiretroviral medications in a sample of patients with human immunodeficiency virus infection. *American Journal of Medicine* 2003; **114**: 573–80.

96 Harwood R, Fountain D, Livermore G. *The Economic Costs of Alcohol and Drug Abuse in the United States, 1992. Report prepared for the National Institute on Drug Abuse and National Institute on Alcohol Abuse and Alcoholism*. NIH Publication No. 98-4327. Rockville, MD: National Institutes of Health; 1998.

97 Grant B, Stinson F, Dawson D *et al*. Prevalence and co-occurrence of substance use disorders and independent mood and anxiety disorders: results from the National Epidemiologic Survey on Alcohol and Related Conditions. *Archives of General Psychiatry* 2004; **61**: 807–16.

98 Hasin D, Stinson F, Ogburn E *et al.*, op. cit.

99 Fernandez A, Marlatt G, Begley E. Family and peer interventions for adults: past approaches and future directions. *Psychology of Addictive Behaviors* 2006; **20**: 207–13.

100 Stanton M. Getting reluctant substance abusers to engage in treatment/self-help: a review of outcomes and clinical options. *Journal of Marital and Family Therapy* 2004; **30**: 165–82.

101 Miller P, Ornstein S, Nietert P *et al*. Self-report and biomarker alcohol screening by primary care physicians: the need to translate research into guidelines and practice. *Alcohol and Alcoholism* 2004; **39**: 325–8.

102 Bradley K, Curry S, Koepsell T *et al*. Primary and secondary prevention of alcohol problems: U.S. internist attitudes and practices. *Journal of General Internal Medicine* 1995; **10**: 67–72.

103 Spandorfer J, Israel Y, Turner B. Primary care physicians' views on screening and management of alcohol abuse: inconsistencies with national guidelines. *Journal of Family Practice* 1999; **48**: 899–902.

104 National Institute on Alcohol Abuse and Alcoholism. *Helping Patients with Alcohol Problems*. NIH Publication No. 03-3769. Bethesda, MD: National Institute on Alcohol Abuse and Alcoholism; 2003.

105 American Psychiatric Association. *Diagnostic and Statistical Manual of Mental Disorders, Fourth Edition (DSM-IV)*. Washington, DC: American Psychiatric Association; 1994.

106 Taj N, Devera-Sales A, Vinson D. Screening for problem drinking: does a single question work? *Journal of Family Practice* 1998; **46:** 328–35.

107 Allen J, Wilson V, eds. *Assessing Alcohol Problems: a guide for clinicians and researchers.* 2nd edn. Bethesda, MD: National Institute on Alcohol Abuse and Alcoholism, US Department of Health and Human Services, Public Health Service; 2007.

108 Graham A, Schultz T, Mayo-Smith M *et al*. *Principles of Addiction Medicine*. 3rd edn. Chevy Chase, MD: American Society of Addiction Medicine, Inc.; 2003.

109 Ewing J. Detecting alcoholism: the CAGE questionnaire. *Journal of the American Medical Association* 1984; **252:** 1905–7.

110 Dhalla S, Kopec J. The CAGE questionnaire for alcohol misuse: a review of reliability and validity studies. *Clinical and Investigative Medicine* 2007; **30:** 33–41.

111 National Institute on Alcohol Abuse and Alcoholism, op. cit.

112 National Institute on Alcohol Abuse and Alcoholism. *Helping Patients Who Drink Too Much: a clinician's guide*. NIH Publication No. 05-3769. Bethesda, MD: National Institute on Alcohol Abuse and Alcoholism; 2005.

Helping alcohol-dependent and problem drinkers to abstain

113 Bayard M, McIntyre J, Hill K *et al*. Alcohol withdrawal syndrome. *American Family Physician* 2004; **69:** 1443–50.

114 Ibid.

115 Kaskutas L. Alcoholics Anonymous effectiveness: faith meets science. *Journal of Addictive Diseases* 2009; **28:** 145–57.

116 Chappel J, Dupont, R. Twelve-step and mutual-help programs for addictive disorders. *Psychiatric Clinics of North America* 1999; **22:** 426–2.

117 Alcoholics Anonymous. *Comments on A.A.'s Triennial Surveys*. New York: Alcoholics Anonymous World Services, Inc.; 1989.

118 Institute of Medicine. *Broadening the Base of Treatment for Alcohol Problems*. Washington, DC: National Academies Press; 1990.

119 Valliant G. *The Natural History of Alcoholism Revisited*. Cambridge, MA: Harvard University Press; 1995.

120 Alcoholics Anonymous. *The Big Book of Alcoholics Anonymous*. 4th edn. New York: Alcoholics Anonymous World Services, Inc.; 2001.

121 Kaskutas L, op. cit.

122 Bandura A. *Social Learning Theory*. Morristown, NJ: General Learning Press; 1971.

123 Kaskutas L, op. cit.

124 Laudet A, Morgen K, White W. The role of social supports, spirituality, religiousness, life meaning and affiliation with 12-step fellowships in quality of life satisfaction among individuals in recovery from alcohol and drug problems. *Alcoholism Treatment Quarterly* 2006; **24:** 33–73.

125 Kelly J, Myers M, Brown S. Do adolescents affiliate with 12-step groups? A multivariate process model of effects. *Journal of Studies on Alcohol and Drugs* 2002; **63**: 293–304.

126 Zemore S. A role for spiritual change in the benefits of 12-step involvement. *Alcoholism: Clinical and Experimental Research* 2007; **31(Suppl.):** S76–9.

127 Kaskutas L, Bond J, Humphreys K. Social networks as mediators of the effect of Alcoholics Anonymous. *Addiction* 2002; **97:** 891–900.

128 Timko C, Finney J, Moos R. The 8-year course of alcohol abuse: gender differences in social context and coping. *Alcoholism: Clinical and Experimental Research* 2005; **29:** 612–21.

129 Bond J, Kaskutas L, Weisner C. The persistent influence of social networks and Alcoholics Anonymous on abstinence. *Journal of Studies on Alcohol* 2003; **64:** 579–88.

130 Humphreys K, Mankowski E, Moos R *et al*. Do enhanced friendship networks and active coping mediate the effect of self-help groups on substance abuse? *Annals of Behavioral Medicine* 1999; **21:** 54–60.

131 Kelly J, Myers M, Brown S. Do adolescents affiliate with 12-step groups? A multivariate process model of effects. *Journal of Studies on Alcohol* 2002; **63:** 293–304.

132 Morgenstern J, Labouvie E, McCrady B *et al*. Affiliation with Alcoholics Anonymous after treatment: a study of its therapeutic effects and mechanisms of action. *Journal of Consulting and Clinical Psychology* 1997; **65:** 768–77.

133 Timko C, Finney J, Moos R, op. cit.

134 Humphreys K, Mankowski E, Moos R *et al*., op. cit.

Helping a problem drinker who is not an alcoholic to cut down

135 Institute of Medicine. *Broadening the Base of Treatment for Alcohol Problems*. Washington, DC: National Academies Press; 1990.

136 Humphreys K. Alcohol and drug abuse: a research-based analysis of the Moderation Management controversy. *Psychiatric Services* 2003; **54:** 621–2.

137 Kishline A. *Moderate Drinking: the Moderation Management guide for people who want to reduce their drinking*. New York: Crown; 1994.

138 An archive of editorials on the Moderation Management controversy can be found at http://doctordeluca.com/documents/primarydocuments.htm

139 Ibid.

140 Coldwell B, Heather N. Introduction to the special issue. *Addiction Research and Training* 2006; **14:** 1–5.

141 Koerkel J. Behavioural self-management with problem drinkers: one-year follow-up of a controlled drinking group treatment approach. *Addiction Research and Theory* 2006; **14:** 35–49.

142 Coldwell B, Heather N, op. cit.

143 Miller S, Rollnick S. *Motivational Interviewing: preparing people for change*. New York: Guilford; 2002.

144 Rotgers F, Kern M, Hoeltzel R. *Responsible Drinking: a Moderation Management approach for problem drinkers*. Oakland, CA: New Harbinger Publications, Inc.; 2002.

145 Clabby J. Helping depressed adolescents: a menu of cognitive-behavioral procedures

for primary care. *The Primary Care Companion to the Journal of Clinical Psychiatry* 2006; **8:** 131–41.

146 Heather N. Controlled drinking, harm reduction and their roles in the response to alcohol-related problems. *Addiction Research and Theory* 2006; **14:** 7–18.

Managing stress, panic, and depression

UNDERSTANDING STRESS IN TODAY'S WORLD

In 2009, the American Psychological Association commissioned its annual survey of stress in America,[1] questioning 1,568 adults living in the U.S. in 2009. The respondents were men, women, employed, unemployed, white non-Hispanic and black, aged 18 to 64 years or older, and drawn from the East, South, Mid-West, and West. That survey reported the following findings.[2]

Americans perceived stress as peaking in 2008 alongside the daily reports about layoffs, home foreclosures, and the continued effects of the international financial meltdown. Nearly a quarter of Americans had experienced a high stress level in the previous month, reporting a score of 8, 9, or 10 on a 10-point scale,[2] and 25% stated that their stress level had increased over the past year. Less than half of the adults who were told by their healthcare providers to make lifestyle changes recall having been given an explanation for the recommendation (46%) or offered advice or shown techniques to help them to make such changes (35%). There is clearly a need for advisors to fill this void by sharing practical stress management techniques.

The advisor can start by offering an explanation of how the stress response works. It is a healthy self-protection process as the body prepares to successfully confront or avoid danger (i.e. the 'flight or fight' response). When appropriately activated, the stress response prepares people to physically handle such challenges as suddenly avoiding an oncoming automobile, or rescuing a child who is starting to walk into traffic. The brain sends signals to the hormones that propel people into action. Breathing quickens to increase oxygen intake, the heart beats faster, blood pressure rises, muscles tighten, and the senses are then sharper. The problems start when this helpful, full-body, defensive, combative response is repeatedly activated by events that do not require this level of physical action (e.g. answering a phone call, stopping in traffic, or watching news on television). Chronically and unnecessarily becoming physically "charged up" to flee or fight can often result in health problems, including high blood pressure, which is a major risk factor for heart disease. The stress response also suppresses the immune system, and so increases the susceptibility to colds and other illnesses. Stress build-up also contributes to anxiety and depression.[3] Management of stressors prevents the onset of disease, reduces the symptoms of existing disease, prevents relapses in recovered individuals, and minimizes the recurrence of symptoms of diseases that are controlled (e.g. heart disease, depression).

The effectiveness of stress management programs has been well documented for many years now.[4] What are the characteristics of people who handle stress well and who are successful and happy in both their personal and working lives? Research compiled by psychologist Daniel Goleman and others indicates that the answer may lie within the concept now known as *emotional intelligence*.[5] This concept calls attention to the fact that success requires more than intellectual IQ, because conventional markers of intelligence do not take into account essential behavioral and character elements. Most advisors know people who are intellectually brilliant yet socially and inter-personally inept. Possession of a high IQ is not necessarily associated with success in work, family life and friendships. Emotional intelligence is composed of five key elements, namely knowing one's own emotions, managing one's own emotions, motivating oneself, recognizing and understanding other people's emotions, and managing relationships by handling others' emotions. The first two elements of emotional intelligence – knowing and managing one's own emotional state – are the central features of effective stress management. Handling stress begins with recognizing the early warning signs. Advisors can help clients to value and rely upon their personally unique emotional radar system. This could be an internally experienced sign such as breath-holding, muscular tension in the nape of the neck, motor overdrive such as restlessly pacing, the first twinges of a headache, or a mild stomach upset. An external sign might be a supervisor's narrowed and possibly disapproving gaze. Once the client has identified their own unique personal early warning system, they can respond by using the following stress management techniques.

IMAGERY BRINGS PEACE

Stress management techniques help to clear the head so that the client can think more logically and systematically about how to solve problems. The three classic stress management techniques are *imagery*, *breathing*, and *muscle relaxation*, referred to here as IBM as a way to facilitate client recall. They are discussed in that order below.

An advisor can teach clients guided imagery to privately conjure up the details of being in a particularly calming situation, such as a place where the client feels safe and happy. For example, a client might choose to be in a garden on a beautiful sunny summer morning, with warm sunlight gently appearing through the forest, and so on. This stress management tool is one of the world's oldest healing resources.[6] It is estimated that 10 million North Americans of all ages practice some form of imagery or meditation to reduce stress, to boost the immune system, and to deal with serious illnesses. It is a practice that is gaining in popularity, and the number of people practicing imagery has doubled in the last 10 years.[7,8] Over the years, imagery-based relaxation experiences have been successfully used to reduce stress in a wide variety of medical populations,[9] including patients with cancer,[10,11] traumatic head injuries,[12] and chronic pain.[13]

By practicing imagery, the client can become skilled at thinking of a multisensory experience in order to capture an external multi-sensory experience that is not present. The goal is to feel calm, safe, content, happy, and relaxed.[14] For example, a client might choose an image of the ocean, as they find that this reduces stress. They could choose to visualize the color of the ocean, hear the pounding of the surf, feel the brisk cool waves splashing against their feet, smell the sea air, and perhaps taste the salty ocean water.[15]

The advisor can teach the five-image PEACE experience:

➤ Place: imagining a safe and peaceful place.
➤ Exercise: imagining the pleasant muscular let-down feeling after a satisfying physical activity.
➤ Affection: imagining a pleasant experience of love and affection.
➤ Compliment: imagining and recalling a compliment that was particularly meaningful.
➤ Excellence: imagining an experience of performing at an excellent level.

The following is a script that the advisor can use to help the client to experience the stress-reducing effects of PEACE. Note that the language used is deliberately invitational, so as to leave the choice of the details under the control of the client. There are several reasons for this. The client's own imagination can create a more personally powerful and meaningful image than an advisor could provide. If the client wants to share the details of the image, that is fine. At the same time, keeping the details of the image private maintains the personally experienced power of the image. Another reason for avoiding suggesting specific images is that the client's history in relation to that image may not be known. For example, having a client imagine "going to a beautiful Caribbean beach where the sun is warm . . . hearing the sounds of gentle reggae music . . . being near the warm, clear blue water" may be a calming choice for the advisor, but it may inadvertently cause stress for a client who struggles with beach images because these generate body image problems. Or a client might associate a beach image with an interpersonal conflict with a significant other, or even with a robbery or assault. There are many personally relaxing images that clients can tap into, envision, and change over time as they see fit. For example, this personal apothecary of soothing images for one client could include visiting a grandparent's home as a child, or for another client imagining hiking with a close friend on a wooded trail on a crisp autumn day. The advisor uses a peaceful tone of voice to gently facilitate the client imagining the specifics of their own privately held images. In the following script, the advisor also suggests that the client should gently associate a different finger with each image, as a way to kinesthetically remember the image.

Place

"As a way to remember these images, you can associate each one with a different finger. If you want to, you can elevate your first finger ever so slightly, and then if you wish let it rest again. Here, you can if you like . . . imagine a place that for you is a safe . . . pleasant . . . and restful place. You might, in your mind's eye, go there. While you are there in this safe, pleasant, and comfortable place, you can if you wish look around a bit. There may be some colors and shapes of things that you like to see. There may be sounds that remind you of this safe and pleasant place. Some people associate pleasant fragrances with being in such a safe, pleasant, and comfortable place. You might, if you'd like to, imagine what it feels like physically to be in this safe, comfortable, and pleasant place."

Exercise

"Very good. If you'd like, you can elevate the next finger for a moment. You can imagine having successfully completed a really satisfying physical activity or exercise experience. Your muscles have been pleasantly spent and you can let yourself experience that muscle relaxation . . . that nice let-down feeling. This can be appreciated by a wide range of muscle groups . . . your arms, your legs . . . wherever in your body you choose to let relaxation come. That pleasant experience following a satisfying physical activity can be so enjoyable to imagine . . . that soothing feeling of muscular release coming into your body . . . permitting yourself to experience and enjoy those sensations."

Affection

"Great. You can, if you want, elevate the next finger for a moment. Here you can choose, if you like, to recall an affectionate and pleasant loving experience. In that image, you can feel safe and cared for . . . you can permit yourself . . . to have a pleasant recall of that experience . . . one that is so loving and affection-ate for you."

Compliment

"Very nice. Here you can, if you'd like, raise your next finger for a moment. In this image, you might consider when you received and accepted a compliment that meant so much to you . . . perhaps because of who gave you that compliment . . . perhaps because of what was said by this person . . . perhaps because of how you felt on receiving such a meaningful compliment."

Excellence

"OK. If you want, you can gently let all your fingers relax and consider calling up another image. It can be an image of you succeeding in something that was very important to you . . . it could be something regarding your family . . . friends . . . associates at work . . . or at school. You were very proud of the excellent job you did with this. You can go back to re-visit this. Consider, if you wish, what it feels like . . . as you reflect on the pride you may feel."

INTENTIONAL BREATHING

Across cultures and centuries, wise people have encouraged the use of this second component of the IBM approach, namely *intentional breathing*. It is the most portable anti-stress, anti-anxiety medication. The influence of the way in which people breathe on their emotional experience is a commonly known psycho-physiological awareness. Breathing as it relates to stress management is so imbedded in the cultural psyche that some clients could probably recall, recite, or complete comments such as "I need a breath of fresh air", "She breathed a sigh of relief", "So much is happening, let me catch my breath", or "After this argument I need some breathing space."

The maintaining of breathing patterns that were used in stressful situations and that are now no longer needed can initiate or worsen stress. For example, when a person learns to control eye–hand coordination to use a new tool, they will concentrate in order to avoid making errors. Accordingly, they make an effort to keep their body still to avoid making mistakes. This often includes holding their breath. Another example is the way that a person's breathing pattern changes when a burst of energy is needed. They will breathe quickly and shallowly in order to have enough energy to better face up to or escape from a dangerous situation. Consider, for example, how a sudden noise in the middle of the night would startle someone awake. Without thinking, they may suddenly hold their breath, vigilantly scan their immediate surroundings, and be on the alert. The advisor can also bring the client's attention to how breathing changes to reflect life events, such as the grateful sigh once a meeting with a son or daughter's teacher is over.

However, the problem is that many clients have over-learned this rapid shallow breathing for energy or this breath-holding for concentration. They are then conditioned to use the same breathing pattern when they are off duty and no longer need to breathe that way.

Good intentional breathing habits involve effortless abdominal breathing, allowing the breath to move in and out without striving. This approach invokes internal quieting, mindfulness, relaxation, and peripheral warming. People report that abdominal breathing is one of the most useful stress reduction techniques.

The following steps can be used by the advisor when coaching clients to use intentional abdominal breathing. It is important to note that learning to adjust the breathing to facilitate stress reduction will paradoxically initially involve some effort and practice.[16]

Instructions such as the following are important because the advisor can then avoid making casual comments such as "Oh, you might want to try some slow breathing" or "Just take a deep breath, it will really help." That style of instruction, because it is delivered in such a casual and off-handed manner, will give the client the impression that this is an unimportant afterthought, and that their advisor is not really serious about this technique. Advice casually given will be casually received. The advisor should project confidence in the usefulness of intentional breathing to reduce stress, because clients' expectation or belief in what is offered is a powerful change agent. One of the key ideas that the advisor should remember is that the relaxing effect is less about *taking* a deep breath, and more about *letting go of* a deep breath. The advisor can help the client to gently move towards an exhalation that is approximately twice as long as the inhalation. It is this particular motion that appears to facilitate the abdominal or belly breathing that is so physically and psychologically healing. The following guidelines will help the advisor to teach this skill.

The advisor can begin by commenting that before, during, or after a stressful experience people often automatically sigh. This allows them to release the tension and take in more soothing oxygen. The client can start to get control over stress by intentionally breathing out that stress.

The advisor suggests that the client should place one hand on the beltline and the other hand on the chest, in order to observe which parts of the body move as the breath enters and leaves. The advisor models this, as well as the mindful breathing, throughout the practice. Placing the hand on the beltline and chest is used to provide some feedback during the training, not for application in real life. The advisor can suggest that the client should adopt a curious attitude about this traveling of air into, through, and out of the body. Some clients have likened this to an image such as a river of air flowing in and out. The client can gradually notice how the abdomen will get smaller during exhalation and larger during inhalation. The advisor encourages the client not to worry about appearing fat, because the sign of a belly expanding during inhalation actually signals healthy stress-reducing breathing. The advisor, who is again modeling this, instructs the client to exhale completely through the mouth, using pursed lips and making a whooshing sound.

One of the best ways for clients to remember the essence of intentional breathing is to time the breathing in terms of 4, 7, and 8 seconds.[17] The advisor asks the client to inhale slowly and deeply through the nose for about 4 seconds, and suggests that inhaling can be savored as oxygen pleasure.[18] The advisor can also suggest other potentially personally meaningful images, such as smelling a fragrant flower or enjoying the wonderful aroma of some delicious food.

Next, the advisor suggests that the client holds their breath for about 7 seconds. Then they suggest a slow, even, and complete exhalation through the mouth for about 8 seconds. Exhaling through gently pursed lips helps to keep the exhalation even. The advisor can model how comfortably long an exhalation can be. It is helpful if the advisor models by exhaling audibly and noticeably for a second or so longer than the client. In this way, the client gets an idea of the importance of the long exhalation. The advisor can use imagery here, such as a balloon expanding in the abdomen, or experiencing the muscle relaxation feeling as the letting go happens.[19] The advisor should ask the client to identify regular points in the day (e.g. at mealtimes, or when putting on or taking off a seat belt) when abdominal breathing can be practiced and eventually over-learned.

MUSCLE RELAXATION

This final part of the IBM approach relates to muscle relaxation. The father of this approach, Dr. Edmund Jacobsen, said that an anxious mind cannot exist in a relaxed body.[20] Tense, stressed-out, worried and anxious clients can find relief from their distress and the accompanying physical symptoms by learning how to reduce muscle tension. During psychological distress, the body experiences a generalized stress activation response involving multiple central and peripheral systems. When a person learns to calm down one of these systems, such as the muscular system, that system sparks a chain reaction which calms the other sub-systems.[21] One review included all of the relevant randomized controlled trials in this area that were published before 2003.[22] It found that, on the basis of 60 clinical outcome studies, muscle relaxation interventions were as effective as pharmacologic, cognitive, or exposure-based procedures for panic disorder with or without agoraphobia, generalized anxiety disorder, and even dental phobia.

Jacobsen's seminal work in this area involved the tensing and releasing of 16 muscle groups so that clients could recognize the difference between tension and relaxation and then facilitate the more desired state in everyday life.[23] Many experimental studies attest to the clinical effectiveness of abbreviated muscle relaxation therapies for several medical conditions and psychiatric disorders.[24] One of the simplest muscular relaxation strategies to teach is the "Relax My Eyes" technique. Here the advisor suggests relaxation of the muscles in the area that could be covered by a Cap or hat, then the Arms, then the Legs, and finally the Middle (CALM). This technique works so well that the client may sometimes lose track of which body part is the focus. This may be a good sign, indicating that relaxation is occurring. If that happens, the client should start again at the beginning with "Relax my eyes, relax my eyes, relax my eyes." Because the procedure is deliberately redundant and simple, it is also often used at bedtime to help clients to allow their bodies to drift off to sleep. The following script teaches this muscular relaxation technique. It begins with the many muscles included in the Cap area, followed by those in the Arm area, the Legs area, and finally the Middle area. The advisor reads from this script in a soothing and gentle tone, and moves in small increments through the muscle groups, asking the client to think as follows.

1 **Cap:** "Relax my eyes . . . (pause for 3 seconds) . . . Relax my eyes . . . (pause for 3 seconds) . . . Relax my eyes . . . (pause for 3 seconds)."
Then the advisor moves on to the next body part within the "Cap" area: Nose . . . Cheeks . . . Jaw . . . Forehead . . . Scalp . . . Neck.
2 **Arms:** "Relax my fingers . . . (pause for 3 seconds) . . . Relax my fingers . . . (pause for 3 seconds) . . . Relax my fingers . . . (pause for 3 seconds)."
Then the advisor moves on to the next body part within the "Arms" area: Hands . . . Forearms . . . Biceps . . . Shoulders . . . Upper back.
3 **Legs:** "Relax my feet . . . (pause for 3 seconds) . . . Relax my feet . . . (pause for 3 seconds) . . . Relax my feet . . . (pause for 3 seconds)."
Then the advisor moves on to the next body part within the "Legs" area: Ankles . . . Heels . . . Calves . . . Thighs

4 **Middle:** "Relax my stomach . . . (pause for 3 seconds) . . . Relax my stomach . . . (pause for 3 seconds) . . . Relax my stomach . . . (pause for 3 seconds)." Then the advisor moves on to the next body part within the "Middle" area: Lower back . . . Buttocks . . . Chest.

The advisor should point out that the client needs to practice the stress management techniques in order to become skilled in their use. And the practice experience should be pleasant, since after all these are stress-reducing techniques! Clients benefit the most when they practice these techniques when they are not stressed. Once they have over-learned the techniques, they can reliably draw upon them when they sense the early warning signs of stress. This is similar to developing any other new skill, such as a new driver who expects to perform better on the busy highway after first practicing in a quiet residential area. Like driving skills, stress management skills can quickly become a way of life. Practicing does not take up extra time because using these skills can become part of the client's existing daily routine (e.g. before making a phone call, during a meeting at work, or when buckling a car seat belt). And no one else needs to know that this practice is happening, if that is important.

Unfortunately, there may be some cynicism about stress management. For example, a client may think or even say "I already know how to breathe, and evidently it hasn't done me much good so far in reducing my stress, has it?" Some of the techniques have been parodied by the entertainment industry and made to look comedic. Even the advisors who teach such techniques have been parodied by being portrayed in silly outfits, working with eccentric-looking clients who present with equally comical complaints. The well-kept secret is that despite the entertainment industry's clever portrayals, there is a great deal of evidence that such stress management techniques do relieve stress, improve health, can be learned in a dignified way, and are used by many of the world's most successful, hard-nosed, and competitive leaders in business, health, government, service, and professional sports. Clients will benefit from learning more or deeper ways of self-calming with imagery, breathing, and relaxation.

GAINING CONTROL OVER PANIC

Some clients will present with what they describe as a panic attack. Their symptoms may include intense anxiety, rapid heart beat, chest pain, nausea, a sensation of shortness of breath, sweating, shaking, dizziness, and feeling physically trapped. These symptoms could be caused by any number of physical illnesses, so it is important for the client to get a medical check-up for heart, hormonal, and blood sugar issues, especially if the symptoms persist or worsen.

For example, changes in thyroid function can mimic anxiety or panic, and mitral valve prolapse can trigger panic. Changes in estrogen and progesterone can affect the way in which the brain receives neurotransmitters, and when neurotransmitters change, so do physical sensations, mood, thought, and behavior.[25]

If physical illness has been ruled out, the client may be dealing with panic disorder. This is also characterized by repeated and most often unexpected panic attacks followed by a month or more of consistent apprehension about having additional attacks. As with many of the other psychological conditions, care provided by a physician who can prescribe helpful medicine can be instrumental in the successful treatment of individuals with this condition.

The National Institute of Mental Health (NIMH) reports that about 2.7% of people aged 18 years or older have had panic disorder in a given year. This corresponds to approximately 6 million American adults.[26] Panic disorder typically develops in early adulthood, the median age of onset being 24 years, but the age of onset extends throughout adulthood.[27] About one in three people with panic disorder develops agoraphobia, a condition in which the individual becomes fearful of being in any place or situation where escape might be difficult or help unavailable in the event of a panic attack.[28]

For those individuals who would prefer a non-pharmaceutical approach, the American Psychiatric Association[29] recommends cognitive–behavioral therapy (CBT) because of its record of having a positive impact on the experience of panic. The following discussion of the cognitive–behavioral approach assumes that the client has developed a faulty, extremely negative, fatalistic, absolutist habit of thinking about the trigger event (e.g. feeling trapped when eating in a crowded restaurant). The kinds of thoughts that cause and maintain panic disorder include misinterpretations of physical symptoms (e.g. "This must be a heart attack") or misinterpretations of the psychological experience (e.g. "I can't stand this embarrassing feeling that people see me looking this nervous in this restaurant"). The cognitive–behavioral approach targets the thought patterns that maintain the panic. One of the main features of a cognitive–behavioral approach is to discover these faulty beliefs and help the client to vigorously challenge and change them. Clients who have panic disorder also tend to mistakenly underestimate their ability to live through and cope with panic attacks, which commonly last for a minute or so. The CBT-oriented advisor encourages the client to recognize the thoughts that occur during panic attacks, and to consider the evidence for and against these thoughts. When these faulty, exaggerated beliefs have been identified, the advisor and the client review the evidence and generate a more truthful and accurate appraisal of the situation.

Exercise also plays an important role. Provided that the client is healthy enough to exercise regularly, the advisor should recommend this. The evidence suggests that for people who are physically healthy, aerobic exercise such as walking for 60 minutes or running for 20–30 minutes at least four days per week benefits those who have panic symptoms.[30-32] Some clients with panic disorder fear that exercise may provoke an attack, so the advisor should suggest that the client practices some coping strategies first, and then gradually weaves in the exercise portion of the plan.

A major goal of psychoeducation[33] for panic disorder is to convey that panic symptoms result from the body's natural fear response, and are not dangerous. To reinforce this, the advisor can recommend readings to the client[34-36] that reinforce the concepts introduced in the cognitive–behavioral advising approach.

Some advisors teach mindful and intentional breathing to decrease anxiety and interrupt the cycle of panic, although the evidence suggests that this is probably not a necessary component.[37] Yet while mindful breathing is not a critical panic-specific component of treatment, it does feel good, and it has significant face validity, so the advisor may still want to include this.

Self-monitoring is one of the most useful tools for helping clients to gain control over panic. The advisor should ask the client to record daily such information as the trigger, where the panic attack happened, their anxious thoughts, their physical symptoms, the date, time, and location of the event, and importantly the techniques that they used to handle the situation. This information reveals patterns, and this empowers the client to adjust, improve, and solidify effective response strategies.

The symptoms of panic and agoraphobia also result from repeatedly associating the uncomfortable symptoms with the specific trigger. Accordingly, many helpful techniques aim to weaken or eliminate these learned associations. The advisor helps with the corrective learning experiences by strengthening ways to be more calm when in the presence of these triggers. Helping a client to learn self-calming skills and then to practice encountering the dreaded situation armed with techniques strengthens nonanxious responses. Avoiding scary triggers just maintains panic, because this does not give the client opportunities to prove that the situation can be handled. Clients may have internal fear cues such as heart racing or anticipating being embarrassed by having a panic attack and external fear cues such as walking across the supermarket parking lot or being seated at a crowded restaurant where escape is a concern. Exposure to such internal and external cues is necessary to eliminate the panic symptoms, and it is often the most challenging part of the CBT approach. Additional effort on the part of the advisor is often required to motivate the client to begin to encounter difficult exposure situations.

Another element of a successful CBT advising approach is to gradually reduce clients' reliance on safety behaviors such as carrying bottles of aspirin or assuring knowledge of quick routes to the nearest hospital's emergency room. Such safety behaviors often provide the client with an immediate feeling of security. However, they also tend to maintain anxiety in the longer term. Safety behaviors promote the belief that everyday situations such as visiting the supermarket are inherently dangerous. This prevents clients from gaining the maximum benefit from successful exposure to anxiety-provoking situations. Therefore gradual elimination of safety behaviors (e.g. feeling a need to hold onto a supermarket carriage at the food market) is an important goal.

An advisor can suggest to a client the use of a metaphoric image of a wave to help. No matter how powerful a wave may appear to be, it loses its strength, passes quickly, and always disappears. Clients can tell themselves that they can ride over the very temporary feelings of panic just as they can ride over the very temporary ocean wave. The advisor recommends that at the early warning signs of panic, the client should use an easily remembered CBT approach called A WAVE, which is as follows.

Accept. The client should accept that this is indeed a wave of panic. Directly confronting something anxiety-provoking by calling it what it is and giving it a name can be very freeing and help establish some control. The client should therefore call this experience what it is: a panic. The advisor asks "What happens to a wave after it crests? A wave always comes down and gets small . . . always. Like a cresting wave, panic can feel powerful but it is always a very temporary experience." The uncomfortable sensations are always momentary, the client is safe, and this panic experience will end momentarily.

Watch. The client can watch and measure the panic attack in the same way that surfers measure the power of an ocean wave. They should rate this wave of panic on a scale of 0 to 10, where 10 is the strongest and most powerful panic wave ever experienced and 0 is no panic wave at all. Measuring in this way is a cognitive experience. It moves the client away from a more emotional, anxious experience and shifts them towards an intellectual experience. This alone helps to cap the upset feelings and provides greater control.

Act. The client should act by "vigorously talking sense to myself." This involves emphatically and strongly making such self-statements as: "This is not a catastrophe", "I will not die", and "This will pass, it always does" and so on. Believing and being determined that this experience will soon pass and that they will feel back to normal again are very important attitudes for the client to have. The client can also act by mindfully breathing through inhaling deeply through the nose for 4 seconds, holding the breath for 7 seconds, and then letting go of a deep breath for about 8 seconds while visualizing a soothing image.

Video replay. Repeat the AWAVE process from the beginning. Once again the client should accept this experience by calling it a panic wave and watch it again by re-measuring the strength of the panic because the client's anxious feelings will be somewhat weaker because of the actions taken.

Expect that these feelings will continue to weaken within a few moments. The advisor should reiterate that, as uncomfortable as these feelings may seem at one moment, the client will always regain control, and can expect to do so if they use these newly practiced skills.

It is possible that the advisor's efforts may be insufficient to help a client to overcome the panic. In that case it would be important to refer them to a CBT-oriented psychotherapist. Such psychotherapists can invoke a more potent component of CBT by prompting the most common internal fear cues right in the exam room by such techniques as having the client run in place to induce heart pounding, or spinning in a swivel chair. The CBT therapist can also ask the client to breathe through a straw in order to induce dizziness, hyperventilation, light-headedness or shortness of breath. The client can then use the stress reduction techniques during these times. Under the supervision of the therapist, the client performs those exercises repeatedly over a number of sessions until they are no longer fearful of them.

UNIPOLAR DEPRESSION: KNOWING THE MARKERS

It is part of the human condition to feel sad, discouraged, or "down" from time to time. These kinds of feelings usually subside within a day or two. However, a unipolar clinical depression represents a move from discomfort to feeling actual psychological pain. It is a very real, overwhelming, and persistent struggle, and people with this condition cannot just snap out of it. It hinders their working and personal lives. Caring people who know the depressed person well often recognize and feel some level of that tangible pain as well. Unlike sadness, depression is a serious condition and often requires help in the form of support, advice, and medication consultation. It is a growing and costly phenomenon.

By 2020, depression is expected to be the second leading cause of disability worldwide.[38] The price tag of depression in the U.S. is estimated at a staggering $44 billion. This includes $12 billion for the direct costs of treatment, $8 billion in terms of premature death, and $24 billion in terms of absenteeism and diminished effectiveness at work. The true costs are actually much higher, as these figures do not include out-of-pocket family expenses, costs for minor and untreated depression, excessive hospitalizations, general medical services, and diagnostic testing.[39]

An advisor who knows how to systematically identify the symptoms of depression will feel competent and confident. One of the most accurate ways to screen someone for depression is to simply ask the question "Are you feeling depressed?" This common-sense approach should always prevail, so if the client is in tears, the advisor should empathically explore whether this is a passing sadness or a depression. Some clients may be depressed but deny this, because they feel shame about it. The advisor needs to remember the advising basics of creating safety through respectful active listening and looking for an opening in which to gently suggest that depression is a possibility. Clients who are in touch with their feelings, and who feel safe enough to share them, appreciate the opportunity to unburden their pain by talking with the advisor. In turn the advisor can listen to the client's story, offer empathy, provide support, teach strategies to lift the mood, suggest psychotherapy if there is a need for more intense treatment, or recommend a consultation with a physician for a physical exam if some of the symptoms could be signs of a physical illness.

There are some depressed clients whose symptoms emerge in ways that do not signify depression to them, such as losing the ability to concentrate well. Again, if physical illness is ruled out, the advisor can help the client by suggesting that the varied symptoms point to a depression. One method of systematically assessing the presence of such symptoms that point to depression was developed for the use of psychiatry residents at Massachusetts General Hospital by Dr. Cary Gross.[40] He developed a comprehensive assessment known as SIGECAPS, where each letter in the acronym refers to a key diagnostic marker for depression. The eight areas include problems with:

➤ Sleep (either oversleeping or poor sleep)
➤ Interest in pleasurable activities (loss of the capacity to experience pleasure)
➤ Guilt (e.g. feeling worthless, hopeless, or regretful)
➤ Energy (lowered energy levels)
➤ Concentration (loss of the ability to focus)
➤ Appetite (either overeating or loss of appetite)
➤ Psychomotor retardation or agitation
➤ Suicidality.

An additional key element that is important when assessing for unipolar depression is to ask about mood. This factor is included in the screen introduced here as MR SAM'S ICE, which captures Mood, Regret, Sleep, Appetite, Motor activity, Suicide, Interests, Concentration, and Energy. The advisor can introduce this assessment by using such wording as the following:

"Bob, I'm going to ask you some questions about symptoms you might have. It will help us get a better handle on what is going on. Would that be alright with you?"

Mood: "Bob, from time to time people feel depressed or down or even hopeless. Have you been having any of those feelings lately?"

Regret: "Do you have any strong thoughts or feelings of regret or guilt, like you did something or did not do something and it really disappointed or let you or your family down?"

Sleep: "Some people have trouble sleeping. How about you? Tell me about any difficulty you may have falling asleep, staying asleep, sleeping too much, or waking up on your own too early in the morning."

Appetite: "Have you noticed that your appetite has been changing? Have you been eating too little or too much? Some people have lost a lot of weight or gained a lot of weight even when they were not trying. How about you?"

A positive response in terms of either weight loss or weight gain should prompt the advisor to recommend that the client arranges to have a physical exam.

Motor activity: "Bob, do you notice or have other people noticed you move or speak more slowly than usual? Or have you been very fidgety, or restless, or moving around quite a bit?"

Suicide: "Have you been thinking about committing suicide or otherwise injuring yourself, or killing others?"

Because there should be no ambiguity about this matter, it is important to actually use the words "suicide" and "killing." Some clients who are contemplating suicide will answer "No" to the question "Have you been thinking about hurting yourself?" This is because *not* to attempt suicide, in their view, would be hurtful. Many more people experience suicidal thoughts than actually attempt suicide, so while it is standard practice to ask about suicidal thoughts, this is not a robust indicator.[41] The advisor should add two further questions that are superior in ascertaining risk for suicide. The first question relates to ascertaining whether there is psychic pain in which the client feels disconnected, empty, or worthless. The second question concerns whether the client feels hopeless, is not seeing the situation getting better, or feels that life is not worth living.[42,43] The advisor should also ask whether the client has a specific plan and has access to such deadly means as firearms. If the advisor senses a risk for suicide, even if the responses to the other assessment questions are negative, the client should be diagnosed as having a major depression. Suicidal thoughts trump all other screening questions. The client should go to the Emergency Department of the nearest hospital, where the medical staff can assess them for possible medication management and/or inpatient treatment.

Assuming that the client is not at risk for suicide, the next assessment question is as follows:

> **Interests:** "Bob, have you been losing interest in the things and activities that used to make you happy . . . that were fun for you . . . or used to give you pleasure?"
>
> **Concentration:** "Are you having trouble focusing and concentrating, such as when you are trying to read, watch television, or work on the computer? Have you been having any significant problems in being able to make decisions?"
>
> **Energy:** "Here's the last question on my list, Bob. How has your energy level been? Are you feeling listless . . . or tired . . . or that you have little energy?"

It is important to note that such depressive disorders often coexist with other disorders such as anxiety disorder, and substance abuse (including alcohol abuse).[44] The following are brief explanations of the most common clinical depressions that an advisor might see.

Major depression, dysthymia, and postpartum depression

Major depression is also known as *major depressive disorder*. It is disabling and interferes with a person's ability to work, sleep, study, eat, and enjoy activities that were once pleasurable. Major depression may occur only once in a person's lifetime, but more often it recurs at different points in their life. Major depression is indicated if in the same 2 weeks there was a change from previous functioning. At least 5 of MR SAM'S ICE were positive for most of the day with at least one element being depressed Mood and/or diminished Interests/pleasure. Major depressive disorder affects approximately 14.8 million American adults, or about 6.7% of the U.S. adult population in a given year.[45] Although it can develop at any age, the median age at onset is 32 years.[46] It is more prevalent in women than in men.[47] Major depressive disorder is actually the leading cause of disability in the U.S. for people aged 15–44 years.[48]

Dysthymia (which is also known as dysthymic disorder) is characterized by an ongoing low-level feeling of depression that is present for most of the day, on most days, for at least 2 years for adults and one year for children. The symptoms are less severe and typically not as disabling as those found in major depression. This disorder affects approximately 1.5% of the U.S. population aged 18 years or older in a given year.[49] This figure is equivalent to about 3.3 million American adults.[50] The median age of onset of dysthymic disorder is 31 years.[51]

Postpartum depression. It is estimated that during the first 3 months after child-birth, 14.5% of women will have a new episode of depression,[52] and 10–20% of mothers are believed to suffer with depression at some time during their post-partum course,[53] which makes postpartum depression the most common serious postpartum disorder.[54] The presence of such maternal depressive symptoms at a critical time for the infant and family has additional adverse effects, such as marital distress,[55] problems with mother–infant interaction and attachment,[56] and adverse behavioral and cognitive effects on the child.[57] Many experts believe that new mothers remain at increased risk for depression for up to 1 year after delivery.[58]

BIPOLAR DEPRESSION: KNOWING THE MARKERS

There are many misconceptions about another form of depression, known as bipolar depression or bipolar disorder. Clients with bipolar depression actually spend much more time being depressed than they spend in the increased-energy episodes known as hypomania, or the extreme-energy episodes known as mania. Accordingly, bipolar depression often goes undiagnosed by health-care professionals, and is often misdiagnosed as a unipolar depression because the high-voltage behaviors of mania just do not occur nearly as often as the depressed mood. Furthermore, the client may not complain about the manic behaviors. This is because such experiences can feel good at the time, although they often eventually lead to behaviors that damage relationships at home and at work and even violate the law. It is critically important for the advisor to assess clients who report feeling depressed for bipolar depression, because any client with this disorder should be referred to a health professional who is skilled in prescribing mood-stabilizing medications.

There are two major kinds of bipolar depression, namely bipolar I and bipo-lar II disorder.

Bipolar I disorder is characterized by dramatic behaviors that may result in a person losing their job, getting into fights, or somehow coming to the atten-tion of the police or authorities. It involves a high-octane, high risk-taking, and dangerous state of mania. For a minority of these bipolar I clients, it may even involve a psychotic, deluded break with reality. Again, because the actual amount of time a bipolar client spends in the manic phase is so small, it unfortunately often takes years for health professionals to accurately diagnose this condition. Hospitalization often helps these clients to stabilize and get better.

Bipolar II disorder is much more common. When a client is hypomanic, this may be experienced as being in a really good mood. During hypomanic episodes they may be more talkative than usual, playful, have increased energy, and be more productive, and may also become involved in high-risk activities that can have psychologically painful consequences.

To make an accurate assessment, the advisor may need to question the client's family members and friends. Hypomania can feel good to the client, who may be oblivious to the impact that it is having on family and work life. A client who is in a manic or hypomanic phase may describe the experience as "I feel as though I am capable of anything and everything" or "This can be an amazing sensation, but I can also get frustrated and angry with others", or "My ideas flow constantly and at high speed. It's as if my brain is in overdrive." People do not complain about feeling good. It is more likely that the client will be a family member or friend who has come to talk about the dangerous or risky nature of some of the more high-voltage episodes. Furthermore, a client with bipolar I disorder may simply not be able to remember the extreme behavior that they engaged in during the troubling manic episodes.

Medicines are regarded as the first line of treatment for bipolar depression, which is a most serious condition. The medicines such as fluoxetine (Prozac), which are often used to treat unipolar depression, are used very carefully by specialist physicians (e.g. psychiatrists), because these medicines can actually trigger a manic episode. It is currently recommended that such antidepressants only be used for short periods of time during severe episodes of depression, and that they be combined with mood-stabilizing medicines.[59]

Although pharmacological interventions remain the primary treatment approach, psychosocial interventions are also important. Such treatment focuses on critical elements that pharmacology cannot address. This includes encouraging the client to take a more active role in self-management, such as taking their medicines properly, understanding their illness, noticing the early warning signs of symptoms, and developing important stress management skills.[60–64] Often the involvement of family and/or friends in treatment is helpful. They can help the bipolar patient to notice the early warning signs that symptoms are starting to develop, and encourage the patient to take their medicine.

According to the National Institute of Mental Health, bipolar depression is not uncommon. It affects approximately 5.7 million American adults, or about 2.6% of the U.S. population aged 18 years or older in a given year.[65] The median age of onset for bipolar depression is 25 years.[66] Because of its high prevalence, the advisor needs to be able to competently screen for this condition. To do this, they need to ascertain whether hypomanic episodes are occurring. The advisor can then determine whether these episodes are reaching more manic levels. The DIGFAST approach[67,68] is a simple, memorable, and practical assessment tool that refers to the following domains.

➤ **Distractibility:** This has been regarded as possibly the most common symptom of bipolar depression. Is the client poorly focused and engaging in an unusual level of multi-tasking?

➤ **Insomnia:** In unipolar depression, the client has low energy and difficulty in sleeping. In bipolar depression, the client has high energy and requires less sleep. So the advisor should ask whether the client has had episodes of feeling a decreased need for sleep (e.g. feeling rested even after only 3 hours of sleep).

➤ **Grandiose thinking:** Approximately 60% of all manic clients report feelings of omnipotence – that they feel almost god-like in their ability, or that they have celebrity-level status. The advisor should find out to what extent the client displays an unusually inflated sense of personal capability.

➤ **Flight of ideas:** Does the client display a thought pattern in which the ideas race on endlessly one after another?

➤ **Activities:** Is there an increase in the intensity and pursuit of goal-directed activities such as sexual behavior, work, or school-related tasks? This may be manifested as a psychomotor agitation.

➤ **Speech:** Does the client seem to talk incessantly and only occasionally come up for air, giving others little chance to talk? Do they seem pressured to produce a fast flow of words? Is it as if the thoughts flow directly from the brain to the tongue without cognitive filtering?

➤ **Thoughtlessness:** This is characterized by the client's inability to anticipate the real-life consequences of their actions, and it leads to an increase in risk-taking behaviors. This unfortunate quality gives rise to excessive involvement in the kind of pleasurable activities that can have painful consequences (e.g. abusing substances, gambling, extravagant spending sprees, making foolish and reckless financial investments, and sexual indiscretions).

MANAGING UNIPOLAR DEPRESSION

Antidepressant medication and psychotherapy have been shown to be equally effective for treating moderate or severe major depression.[69,70] Although some medicines can help with unipolar depressions, many clients are concerned about the ongoing cost, the delayed effectiveness of the drugs, interaction with other drugs, and the potential side-effects of these medicines. There are practical, non-pharmaceutical treatments that can be offered along with the medicine or in place of it.

The practical lifestyle suggestions described here for unipolar depression come from the evidence-based heritage of CBT. The following framework can be used to organize an effective way of responding. Inspired by John Christensen's SPEAK approach,[71,72] it is organized as the BE FAST technique – Bravery, Exercise, Fun, Act, Solve, and Think.[73] The advisor can choose one, several, or all elements of the BE FAST menu to introduce mood-enhancing techniques. Cognitive therapy approaches, such as BE FAST, can be as effective as medications for the initial management of moderate or severe depression, with the level of impact relating to the advisor's level of experience or competence.[74] Not only has cognitive therapy such as a BE FAST approach been shown to be as effective as medication, but also such CBT approaches have an enduring impact that extends beyond the end of treatment.[75] The BE FAST approach can be summarized as follows.

➤ **Bravery:** The advisor encourages the client to act in increasingly brave ways by sharing their thoughts and feelings with others. This increases their energy and improves their mood. Repressing one's feelings and thoughts is hard work, and it drains one's energy. However, speaking with others divides the sorrows and multiplies the joys. This bravery element of BE FAST relates to being appropriately assertive. The advisor should recommend that clients take calculated risks by standing up for themselves and stating what they want to have happen. It also refers to encouraging clients to express their positive feelings as well (e.g. expressing gratitude to others), an equally important part of being brave. Clients can start to reveal a bit more about their thoughts and feelings to people whom they already trust. They can begin to increase the level of what they share, and reveal a little more about themselves. The advisor should compliment the client for their bravery in sharing their story with the advisor.

➤ **Exercise:** A review of 25 randomized controlled clinical trials indicated that exercise alleviates the symptoms of depression, and that maintaining the exercise over time maintains the positive emotional effects.[76] Many people can begin to feel these positive effects with moderate exercise such as a 20-minute walk taken three times per week. Working out does not have to be the laborious experience that intimidates some clients, such as choosing, paying for, and committing to a gym, having to buy special exercise shoes and clothes, and perspiring profusely, as well as the potentially inhibiting planning that is necessary. Simply taking walks will be very effective.

➤ **Fun:** The advisor can ask the client to remember those fun, healthy things that they used to do when they were not depressed. This does not by any means have to be at the level of taking an expensive vacation. It is mostly about the inexpensive, everyday available activities, such as calling a good friend who has not been heard from for a while, playing some upbeat music, or watching a favorite comedy on television.

➤ **Act:** The advisor should urge the client to act on the elements of BE FAST even if they do not feel up to it. If a client who feels depressed decides to wait until their mood improves before they act on this BE FAST list, they may be waiting for a long time – and stunting their emotional self. The client who starts to implement the elements of BE FAST will find that their actions result in a more positive mood.

➤ **Solve:** The advisor should remind the client that they have already been able to solve significant life problems, and should encourage them to respect that reality. Accomplishing what they have already achieved will have necessitated some out-of-the-box thinking. The advisor should tell the client that they never have to feel stuck, because there are always a number of healthy solutions. Helping the client to embrace their identity as a problem solver is very important. The advisor can teach the client to remember that successful problem solvers describe the problem, name how they feel, identify one goal, and then think of as many solutions as possible to get to that goal.

➤ **Think sensibly:** The advisor should call attention to how clients describe life's events to themselves, as this has much to do with how they feel. It is important that clients choose to perceive what is happening in accurate and therefore healthy ways. Simply put, the brain believes what the client says to it. Therefore the client should be alert in order to avoid quickly making negative, self-bullying self-statements such as "This is . . . awful/terrible/a catastrophe/the last straw", "It always happens to me", or "I can't stand this." This is a form of self-bullying that exacerbates the injury that the client may have already experienced.

A final intervention is to encourage the client to write down or keep a typewritten record of what they are thinking and feeling on a regular basis. This action elevates the mood. This has been demonstrated by a study in which one group of clients was randomly assigned to write one journal entry per day for three days describing an upsetting event. Another group of clients was randomly assigned to a control intervention of casual content writing, also for three days. The clients who wrote about the upsetting events had impressive outcomes, such as having lower physical illness symptom levels at 3-month follow-up, and reported having made fewer visits to their doctors during the 3-month and 15-month follow-up.[77]

REFERENCES
Understanding stress in today's world

1 American Psychological Association. *Stress in America*. Washington, DC: American Psychological Association; 2009.

2 Ibid.

3 Harvard Women's Health Watch. *Breath Control Helps Quell Errant Stress Response*. Boston, MA: Harvard Health Publications; 2006.

4 Iglesias S, Azzara M, Squillace M *et al*. A study on the effectiveness of a stress management programme for college students. *Pharmacy Education* 2005; **5**: 27–31.

5 Goleman D. *Emotional Intelligence: why it can matter more than IQ*. New York: Bantam Books; 1995.

Imagery brings peace

6 Achterberg J. *Imagery in Healing*. Boston, MA: Shambhala; 1985.

7 Trakhtenberg E. The effects of guided imagery on the immune system: a critical review. *International Journal of Neuroscience* 2008; **118**: 839–55.

8 O'Donnell J, Maurice S, Beattie T. Emergency analgesia in the paediatric population. Part III. Non-pharmacological measures of pain relief and anxiolysis. *Emergency Medicine Journal* 2002; **19**: 195–7.

9 Johnson E, Lutgendorf S. Contributions of imagery ability to stress and relaxation. *Annals of Behavioral Medicine* 2001; **23**: 273–81.

10 Walker L, Walker M, Ogston K *et al*. Psychological, clinical, and pathological effects of relaxation training and guided imagery during primary chemotherapy. *British Journal of Cancer* 1999; **80**: 262–8.

11 Wallace K. Analysis of recent literature concerning relaxation and imagery interventions for cancer pain. *Cancer Nursing* 1997; **20**: 79–87.

12 Lysaght R, Bodenhammer E. The use of relaxation training to enhance functional outcomes in adults with traumatic head injuries. *American Journal of Occupational Therapy* 1990; **44**: 787–802.

13 Syrjala K, Abrams J. Hypnosis and imagery in the treatment of pain. In: Gatchel R, Turk D, eds. *Successful Approaches to Pain Management: a practitioner's handbook*. New York: Guilford Press; 1996. pp. 231–58.

14 Roffe L, Schmidt K, Ernst E. A systematic review of guided imagery as an adjuvant cancer therapy. *Psycho-Oncology* 2005; **14**: 607–17.

15 Johnson E, Lutgendorf S, op. cit.

Intentional breathing

16 Conrad A, Muller S, Doberenz S *et al*. Psychophysiological effects of breathing instructions for stress management. *Applied Psychophysiology and Biofeedback* 2007; **32**: 89–98.

17 Weil A. *Breathing: the master key to self-healing – 8 techniques to revitalize your health*. Boulder, CO: Sounds True, Inc.; 1999.

18 Young S. *Break Through Pain: a step-by-step mindfulness meditation program for transforming chronic and acute pain*. Boulder, CO: Sounds True, Inc.; 2004.

19 Ibid.

Muscle relaxation

20 Jacobsen E. *Progressive Muscular Relaxation: a physiological and clinical investigation of muscular states and their significance in psychology and medical practice*. Chicago: University of Chicago Press; 1974.

21 Conrad A, Roth W. Muscle relaxation therapy for anxiety disorders: it works but how? *Journal of Anxiety Disorders* 2007; **21:** 243–64.

22 Jorm A, Christensen H, Griffiths K *et al*. Effectiveness of complementary and self-help treatments for anxiety disorders. *Medical Journal of Australia* 2004; **181(Suppl.):** S29–46.

23 McCallie M, Blum C, Hood C. Progressive muscular relaxation. *Journal of Human Behavior in the Social Environment* 2006; **13:** 51–66.

24 Conrad A, Roth W, op. cit.

Gaining control over panic

25 Wehrenberg M. *The Ten Best-Ever Anxiety Management Techniques: understanding how your brain makes you anxious and what you can do to change it*. New York: WW Norton; 2008.

26 Kessler R, Chiu W, Demler O *et al*. Prevalence, severity, and comorbidity of 12-month DSM-IV disorders in the National Comorbidity Survey Replication. *Archives of General Psychiatry* 2005; **62:** 617–27.

27 Kessler R, Berglund P, Demler O *et al*. Lifetime prevalence and age-of-onset distributions of DSM-IV disorders in the National Comorbidity Survey Replication. *Archives of General Psychiatry* 2005; **62:** 593–602.

28 Robins L, Regier D, eds. *Psychiatric Disorders in America: the Epidemiologic Catchment Area Study*. New York: The Free Press; 1991.

29 American Psychiatric Association. *Practice Guideline for the Treatment of Patients with Panic Disorder*. 2nd edn. Washington, DC: American Psychiatric Association; 2009.

30 Broman-Fulks J, Berman M, Rabian B *et al*. Effects of aerobic exercise on anxiety sensitivity. *Behaviour Research and Therapy* 2004; **42:** 125–36.

31 Stathopoulou G, Powers M, Berry A *et al*. Exercise interventions for mental health: a quantitative and qualitative review. *Clinical Psychology: Science and Practice* 2006; **13:** 179–93.

32 Strohle A, Feller C, Onken M *et al*. The acute antipanic activity of aerobic exercise. *American Journal of Psychiatry* 2005; **162:** 2376–8.

33 American Psychiatric Association, op. cit.

34 Antony MM, McCabe RE. *10 Simple Solutions to Panic: how to overcome panic attacks, calm physical symptoms, and reclaim your life*. Oakland, CA: New Harbinger Publications; 2004.

35 Barlow DH, Craske MG. *Mastery of Your Anxiety and Panic (MAP-3): client workbook for anxiety and panic*. 3rd edn. New York: Oxford University Press; 2005.

36 Ibid.

37 Schmidt NB, Woolaway-Bickel K, Trakowski J *et al.* Dismantling cognitive-behavioral treatment for panic disorder: questioning the utility of breathing retraining. *Journal of Consulting and Clinical Psychology* 2000; **68:** 417–24.

Unipolar depression: Knowing the markers

38 Pignone MP, Gaynes BN, Rushton JL *et al.* Screening for depression in adults: a summary of the evidence for the U.S. Preventive Services Task Force. *Annals of Internal Medicine* 2002; **136:** 765–76.

39 Lam R, Wok H. *Depression.* New York: Oxford University Press; 2008.

40 Carlat D. The psychiatric review of symptoms: a screening tool for family physicians. *American Family Physician* 1998; **58:** 1617–24.

41 Jacobs D, Brewer M, Klein-Benheim M. Suicide assessment: an overview and recommended protocol. In: Jacobs D, ed. *The Harvard Medical School Guide to Suicide Assessment and Intervention.* San Francisco, CA: Jossey-Bass Publishers; 1999. pp. 3–39.

42 Szanto K, Reynolds C, Conwell Y *et al.* High levels of hopelessness persist in geriatric patients with remitted depression and a history of attempted suicide. *Journal of the American Geriatrics Society* 1998; **46:** 1401–6.

43 Jacobs D, Brewer M, Klein-Benheim M, op. cit.

44 Kessler R, Berglund P, Demler O *et al.* Lifetime prevalence and age-of-onset distributions of DSM-IV disorders in the National Comorbidity Survey Replication. *Archives of General Psychiatry* 2005; **62:** 593–602.

45 Kessler R, Chiu W, Demler O *et al.* Prevalence, severity, and comorbidity of 12-month DSM-IV disorders in the National Comorbidity Survey Replication (NCS-R). *Archives of General Psychiatry* 2005; **62:** 617–27.

46 Kessler R, Bergland P, Demler O *et al.*, op. cit.

47 Kessler R, Berglund P, Demler O *et al.* The epidemiology of major depressive disorder: results from the National Comorbidity Survey Replication (NCS-R). *Journal of the American Medical Association* 2003; **289:** 3095–105.

48 World Health Organization. *The World Health Report 2004: Changing History. Annex Table 3: Burden of disease in DALYs by cause, sex, and mortality stratum in WHO regions, estimates for 2002.* Geneva: World Health Organization; 2004.

49 Kessler R, Chiu W, Demler O *et al*, op. cit.

50 US Census Bureau. *Population Estimates by Demographic Characteristics. Table 2: Annual estimates of the population by selected age groups and sex for the United States: April 1, 2000 to July 1, 2004* (NC-EST2004-02). Washington, DC: US Census Bureau; 2005.

51 Kessler R, Berglund P, Demler O *et al.*, op. cit.

52 Gaynes BN, Gavin N, Meltzer-Brody S *et al. Perinatal Depression: prevalence, screening accuracy, and screening outcomes.* Evidence Report/Technology Assessments No. 119. Rockville, MD: Agency for Healthcare Research and Quality; 2005.

53 Steiner M. Perinatal mood disorders: position paper. *Psychopharmacology Bulletin* 1998; **34:** 301–6.

54 Gjerdingen D, Yawn M. Postpartum depression screening: importance, methods, barriers,

and recommendations for practice. *Journal of the American Board of Family Medicine* 2007; **20**: 280–88.

55 Beck CT. Predictors of postpartum depression: an update. *Nursing Research* 2001; **50**: 275–85.

56 Righetti-Veltema M, Bousquet A, Manzano J. Impact of postpartum depressive symptoms on mother and her 18-month-old infant. *European Child and Adolescent Psychiatry* 2003; **12**: 75–83.

57 Grace SL, Evindar A, Stewart DE. The effect of postpartum depression on child cognitive development and behavior: a review and critical analysis of the literature. *Archives of Women's Mental Health* 2003; **6**: 263–74.

58 Gaynes BN, Gavin N, Meltzer-Brody S *et al.*, op. cit.

Bipolar depression: Knowing the markers

59 Sachs GS, Koslow CL, Ghaemi SN. The treatment of bipolar depression. *Bipolar Disorders* 2000; **2**: 256–60.

60 Beynon S, Soares-Weiser K, Woolacott N *et al*. Psychosocial interventions for the prevention of relapse in bipolar disorder: systematic review of controlled trials. *British Journal of Psychiatry* 2008; **192**: 5–11.

61 Scott J. Cognitive therapy as an adjunct to medication in bipolar disorder. *British Journal of Psychiatry* 2001; **178(Suppl.)**: S164–8.

62 Ghaemi SN, Pardo TB, Hsu DJ. Strategies for preventing the recurrence of bipolar disorder. *Journal of Clinical Psychiatry* 2004; **65(Suppl. 10)**: 16–23.

63 Vieta E, Colom F. Psychological interventions in bipolar disorder: from wishful thinking to an evidence-based approach. *Acta Psychiatrica Scandinavica* 2004; **110(Suppl.)**: 34–8.

64 Vieta E. The package of care for patients with bipolar depression. *Journal of Clinical Psychiatry* 2005; **66(Suppl. 5)**: 34–9.

65 Kessler R, Chiu W, Demler O *et al*. Prevalence, severity, and comorbidity of 12-month DSM-IV disorders in the National Comorbidity Survey Replication. *Archives of General Psychiatry* 2005; **62**: 617–27.

66 Kessler R, Berglund P, Demler O *et al*. Lifetime prevalence and age-of-onset distributions of DSM-IV disorders in the National Comorbidity Survey Replication. *Archives of General Psychiatry* 2005; **62**: 593–602.

67 Carlat D. The psychiatric review of symptoms: a screening tool for family physicians. *American Family Physician* 1998; **58**: 1617–24.

68 Gianakos D. The 15-minute visit: when to suspect bipolar disorder. *Patient Care: The Journal of Best Clinical Practices for Today's Physician*. 2007; **January 1**: 1–2.

Managing unipolar depression

69 Cuijpers P, van Straten A, van Oppen P *et al*. Are psychological and pharmacologic interventions equally effective in the treatment of adult depressive disorders? A meta-analysis of comparative studies. *Journal of Clinical Psychiatry* 2008; **69**: 1675–85.

70 Imel ZE, Malterer MB, McKay KM *et al.* A meta-analysis of psychotherapy and medication in unipolar depression and dysthymia. *Journal of Affective Disorders* 2008; **110**: 197–206.

71 Cole S, Christensen J, Raju M *et al.* Depression. In: Feldman M, Christensen J, eds. *Behavioral Medicine in Primary Care: a practical guide.* Stamford, CT: Appleton and Lange; 1997. pp. 187–207.

72 Clabby J, Howarth D. Managing CHF and depression in an elderly patient: being open to collaborative care. *Family, Systems, and Health* 2007; **25**: 457–64.

73 Clabby J. Helping depressed adolescents: a menu of cognitive-behavioral procedures for primary care. *The Primary Care Companion to the Journal of Clinical Psychiatry* 2006; **8**: 131–41.

74 DuRubeis R, Hollon S, Amsterdam J *et al.* Cognitive therapy vs. medications in the treatment of moderate to severe depression. *Archives of General Psychiatry* 2005; **62**: 409–16.

75 Hallon S, DeRubeis R, Shelton R *et al.* Prevention of relapse following cognitive therapy vs. medications in moderate to severe depression. *Archives of General Psychiatry* 2005; **62**: 417–22.

76 Mead G, Morley W, Campbell P *et al.* Exercise for depression. *Cochrane Database of Systematic Reviews* 2009; **Issue 3**: CD004366. DOI: 10.1002/14651858.CD004366.pub4.

77 Gidron Y, Duncan E, Lazar A *et al.* Effects of guided written disclosure of stressful experiences on clinic visits and symptoms in frequent clinic attenders. *Family Practice* 2002; **19**: 161–6.

Marriages, relationships, children, and teens

HELPING TROUBLED MARRIAGES AND RELATIONSHIPS

There is increasing evidence that clients who have a satisfying marriage or relationship are not only happy but are better insulated from harm. For adults, a stable, happy marriage is actually one of the best protectors against illness and premature death. For children, being raised in a family with a stable, happy marriage is the best source of emotional stability and good physical health.[1,2] For example, the incidence of emergency visits for childhood asthma attacks actually increases in direct proportion with tenuous and distant parental relationships (e.g. from married to cohabiting to not living together).[3] Marital discord and conflict between parents is a better predictor of later-life illness for children than the actual marital status of their parents.[4] For women, poor relationship quality is associated with an increased risk of premature mortality and heart disease.[5–8] Married men show improved health status, a decrease in negative physical symptoms, and an increase in positive behaviors for the most part compared with their unmarried peers.[9]

Developing a stable, happy marriage or relationship does not come easily. Statistically, 40% of first marriages, 60% of second marriages, and 73% of third marriages end in divorce.[10] About 75% of those who divorce will eventually remarry.[11] And people remarry quickly – on average, within 4 years of their divorce, and 30% remarry within 1 year.[12] An advisor who is aware of such social trends and is informed by the growing science about successful marriages can make a tremendous impact.

A cultural context that merits consideration is that for many clients, work may be becoming a haven from home life.[13] Home can be a lonely place even if others are there. It can be a noisy interlude with yelling children, an unhappy partner, bills to pay, and household chores to be done. Unlike work, it is hard to standardize one's home life. And in an increasingly money-driven culture, the demands of work financially overshadow what needs to be done at home. The workplace has social gatherings, incentives for working harder, recognition, and, most importantly, a salary. To establish and maintain a happy, stable marriage, a couple needs to be as ambitious for their own relationship as they are for their economic and career-related well-being. Given this, one of the simplest ideas that an advisor can share is that the client joins the "4 H Club" – schedule Hours together, genuinely Hear each other, generously Help each other, and Hold each other. Failure to attend to these four elements helps to explain what is behind clients' reports of marriages that start out so full of promise and then start to crumble.

There are recommendations that are based upon many studies replicated over the years that come from the laboratory of John Gottman.[14] An advisor who is acquainted with this science will be able to help many clients. One of the studies evaluated 130 couples, who were married within 6 months of the study's onset. These couples represented an even distribution of marital satisfaction on the Marital Adjustment Test. They had no children, and fitted the demographic characteristics of the major ethnic and racial groups in the greater Seattle area. The average age of the wives was 25.4 years and that of the husbands was 26.5 years.[15]

A remarkably comprehensive array of assessments was implemented as follows. Once each year, for 6 years, the marital status of the couples was assessed. Each member of the couple would be connected to instruments that measured their heart rate, blood pressure, and skin conductivity. Even the chairs on which they sat measured fidgeting. It was essentially a kind of lie-detector apparatus. In addition, staff videotaped each individual.

Two independent observers who had been trained in the use of the Specific Affect Coding System (SPAFF) scored the participants for facial expressions, vocal tone, and actual words, and classified these into such categories as "neutral", "hostile", "avoidant", and "friendly." Before entering the lab, each couple also filled out the Couple's Problem Inventory (CPI), which identifies major sources of conflict. Once in the lab, with two cameras rolling, each couple was asked to discuss one of these hot topics for 15 minutes. After the interaction they viewed the videotape and were asked to recall how they felt during the interaction. They used a rating dial to provide a continuous self-report measure of their emotional evaluation of the marital interaction.

At the end of the 6-year period, there had been 17 divorces among the 130 couples. The mean time period for which the divorced couples had been married was 3 years. There were of course varying levels of happiness among the stable couples.

The research group has replicated this study many times, and became adept at predicting which marriages would end in divorce within 5 years, with over 80% accuracy based on just one 15-minute session. When a follow-up was performed 10 years later, the accuracy level rose to 90%. The implication of this for advisors is that by pinpointing how marriages destabilize, they can help couples to maintain the happiness that they feel at present, and advise couples who are beginning to have difficulties.

Unhappy marriages resemble each other in one overriding way, and the advisor can alert the client to look out for four warning signs, called the Four Horsemen of the Apocalypse. This concept is based upon the ominous four images of Conquest, War, Famine, and Death, described in the Book of Revelation (6:7–8 in the King James Bible).

The new Four Horsemen of the Apocalypse for marriages are Criticism, Defensiveness, Contempt, and Withdrawal (the latter is also known as Stonewalling, and is particularly toxic if done by men). Later research added Belligerence as another destroyer of marriages and relationships. If these four horsemen enter and stay in a client's marriage, they will trample the relationship. The job of the advisor is to explain what the four horsemen look like, so that the client can stop them at the marital gate, or take retaliatory action if they do get in. Success is actually less about whether these destructive forces start to penetrate a relationship, and more about having the tools to banish them once they have been discovered. Advisors should become skilled at identifying such destructive patterns, which are illustrated in the following description of the demise of the marriage of a modern-age Adam and Eve – a marriage that started out with great promise.

Criticism

One of the first facts that the advisor should explain is that *complaining* is actually fine. It is in fact one of the healthiest activities that can occur, as without it things will not change. Expressing anger and disagreement, rather than suppressing the complaint, can make the marriage stronger in the long term. Eve would complain to Adam about his spending. However, the client needs to be careful that complaining does not develop into the first horseman – criticism. When Eve's complaints did not change Adam's spending habits, something damaging began to happen, as Eve escalated to criticism. Complaining relates to a specific behavior, such as Adam's spending of money, whereas criticism relates to attacking the personality (e.g. "You're so irresponsible"). At this point there has been a slip from complaining to criticizing. The client has started to use generalizations and global phrases such as "You never . . ." or "You always . . .". When Eve says "You always think about yourself", she is assaulting Adam and he hears it loud and clear.

Contempt

Now that criticism has muscled into the marriage, the advisor should be alert to the approaching gallop of the second horseman – contempt. By their first anniversary, this couple had still not resolved their financial differences. Eve was feeling disgusted.

Eve (shrieking):	"Why are you so irresponsible?"
Adam (fed up and insulted):	"Oh shut up. You're so freaking cheap. I don't know how I ended up with you anyway."

Contempt has just entered their relationship. This is the intention to insult one's partner. With words and body language, the client throws insults, uses hostile humor, mocks, and rolls their eyes. Fueling these actions are negative thoughts about the partner – that they are stupid, incompetent, a fool. The client is now having a difficult time remembering a single positive quality or act. Contempt is the roughest of all the four horsemen.

Defensiveness

Once they had allowed contempt to gallop into their home, Adam and Eve's marriage went from bad to worse. When either of them acted contemptuously, the other responded defensively. They each felt victimized by the other, and neither was willing to take responsibility for contributing to their problems. In effect they both constantly pleaded innocent. Examples of the ways in which a partner will deny responsibility include protests (e.g. "I am not to blame"), making excuses, coming up with a counter-complaint, and just repeating their denial. When such patterns emerge in the story, the advisor should help the client to understand the importance of acknowledging a personal mistake or error to their partner. When so much psychological energy is spent convincing one's partner of an error, there is often little energy left over for doing some problem solving.

Withdrawal (also known as stonewalling)

Exhausted and overwhelmed by Eve's attacks, Adam eventually stopped responding and decided not to engage and participate. Instead of arguing, the situation degenerated into Eve screaming at Adam that he was shutting her out: "You never say anything. You just sit there. It's like talking to a brick wall." Stonewalling often happens while a couple is in the process of talking things out. Stonewallers do not seem to realize the devastating effects of this action. While it often has a quiet and non-destructive exterior appearance, withdrawal conveys an icy distance, a smugness, and a hurtful disapproval. As the behaviors of these four horsemen become more entrenched, the couple begins to focus on the escalating negativity and tension. Eventually they become deaf to each other's efforts at peacemaking. While it is hurtful if either partner engages in withdrawal, it is particularly destructive if the man does it.

The advisor will encounter three different overall ways in which couples communicate their differences, namely validating, volatile, and conflict-avoiding. The validating couple makes communication a priority. These couples occasionally squabble but usually address their differences before their anger boils over. Rather than engaging in anger matches, these couples choose to disagree by having quick "meetings" in which each partner has an opportunity to air their perspective.

The volatile couple is easy to recognize because it is literally easy to hear them. They tend to interrupt each other and energetically defend their own point of view rather than listen to what their partner was expressing. Conflict and passionate disputes often erupt. Eventually, however, they reach some sort of agreement.

The conflict-avoiding couple would say that they are on the same page about most things, that they think alike, and that they quickly felt at ease with each other from the beginning. When tension arises, this kind of couple very rarely fights. They might, for example, consider time alone more helpful than talking things out or arguing. These couples rarely confront their differences head on.

While popular lore might argue that one of these marital arrangements is more likely to lead to happiness than the others, the truth is that any of them can characterize a really happy marriage. The advisor can reassure the client about this. A couple can get as mad as they want at each other, or avoid conflict altogether. The key is that the ratio of positive comments and acts to negative comments and acts is 5 to 1 in successful marriages and 15 to 1 in outstanding marriages.

The following is a Sweet Sixteen list of practical recommendations, drawn from the findings of Gottman's research,[16] which the advisor can share with clients.

1 Try to manage, not cure, the inevitable perpetual problems

Over 60% of marital problems are not solved, but managed. The conflict is not about the topic being discussed, but about some underlying deep belief that one partner feels cannot be compromised. The happy couple recognizes that such problems will never be solved, so they avoid the futility of trying to fix them. Rather they manage the perpetual problem. Clients should recognize that such an issue will probably always be with them; they will talk about it, occasionally make some progress, or make the situation better for a short time. Successful couples accept that the problem will probably re-emerge. Such perpetual problems are probably inevitable. It is a rare couple that does not have one. The smart couple adapts to their particular persistent problem rather like a person who has learned to manage a chronic illness.

2 It's not the fight, it's the recovery after a fight that's important

Although many couples would prefer to avoid fights, the fighting in and of itself is not the problem. What is important is the self-soothing after the fight is over. It is critical for the client to bounce back and engage with their partner, rather than becoming sulky or quietly passive. Disagreements between partners are unavoidable. The couple should focus on what helps them to recover from disagreements. A healthy relationship is characterized by one person having the maturity to make a bid to end the argument, and the other person having the maturity to accept the bid.

3 Complaining and feedback are OK

One way for a client to complain to a partner is to name a feeling, briefly describe the problem, and then state the personal goal (e.g. "I feel worried . . . because work seems to take up so much of our time . . . what I'd like is to talk to you more"). Another way of expressing a point of view is for the client to provide feedback by describing the facts of what they have observed, how they feel about it, and their sense of what might happen if this were to continue (e.g. "I notice that work seems to take up so much of our time. . . . I'm worried about that for us . . . because if it continues it won't be fun and we'll also have a hard time figuring out how to handle the kids").

4 Admit your mistakes

If a client in a marriage or relationship is reluctant to admit a mistake, the partner spends valuable energy trying to point this out rather than problem solving. Everyone then loses. To admit a mistake is a sign of confidence and leadership. It allows the couple to move on. If the client who is receiving the feedback wants to respectfully accept the feedback and also express a point of view, the following formula can help. A client can show:

➤ Recognition (e.g. "It's understandable that you would be so upset that I didn't call")

➤ Remorse (e.g. "I'm really sorry that this hurt you so much") *and*

➤ Reason (e.g. "The reason I didn't call was that I didn't want to upset you at work").

Another version of this approach is the See, Sorry, and Say method: "I can See what you are talking about . . . I'm Sorry you are so upset . . . If I can Say what I think happened it might help . . ."

5 Avoid contempt with empathic curiosity

Part of the original attraction that each member of a couple had for each other was a belief that the other person had ideas and beliefs that were appealing. This is important for the client to remember, as it will keep contempt from trampling the relationship. An antidote to contempt is for the client to be sincerely curious about what is behind the partner's point of view. People who are happily married find ways to try to genuinely understand where their partner is coming from. Certainly the client does not have to agree with the partner's perspective, but trying to understand it helps to evict deadly contempt from the home.

6 Engage, and don't withdraw

The advisor should recommend that clients remain strong and engaged in the relationship discussions, agreements, and disagreements. The advisor should tell clients that, so long as physical and psychological safety is not an issue, they can often handle the upset of a disagreement better than they may think. The truth is that when men in particular withdraw or become silent, this is not a benign event. In a heterosexual marriage, this behavior by men has a particularly discouraging effect on the women they care about.

7 Soothe the irritable physiological arousal

Individuals in successful and happy marriages use techniques such as imagery, mindful breathing, muscle relaxation, prayer, appropriate use of humor, and so on to self-calm and soothe their partner. Once agitated, it may take the body about 20 minutes to slow itself down to calm levels. And if a couple uses a time-out to give themselves a break from a disagreement, the man in particular may have to watch a gender-specific tendency to escalate his negative self-talk.

8 Delayed and softened start-up by the female partner

It was found that during 96% of the couples' discussions about hot topics, the tone that was set during the first few minutes of the conversation persisted for a long time. It is important for a couple to keep the first few minutes of their daily encounters positive. The greeting of one another at the end of the working day, and the minutes that follow shortly afterwards, are mood-setting moments. And since it is more often the woman who initiates conversations about problems, she can be advised to delay and soften the start-up. If a small amount of time can first be spent on cultivating a more positive climate, more will be gained from the important discussion to come.

9 A confident man accepts input

Newly married men who accepted input from their wives were the ones who went on to have stable, happy marriages. The advisor should help men to understand this, and that the whole family benefits from a power-sharing relationship. A confident man honors and values his partner's input.

10 Recognize and accept a partner's repair attempts

This is easier to do when there are routinized rituals of everyday encounters where the couple can count on time to connect and bond. The advisor should encourage the client to exercise leadership and make a bid (e.g. smile, give a hug, offer a gentle and disarming joke, or make a cup of tea for the partner). A wise and mature client learns to offer such bids, recognizes them when they are offered, and graciously accepts them.

11 Men should de-escalate the low-intensity negative feelings of their partner

In successful and happy marriages, the man found ways to de-escalate his partner's low-intensity feelings of sadness, anger, whining, tension, fear, and domineering. When she was irritated or whining, he avoided responding in kind. Rather, he found a way to calm both of them down a bit. A smart man attends to and soothes the small irritations of his partner.

12 Women should de-escalate the high-intensity negative feelings of their partner

In happy and successful marriages, the woman learned to help to calm the major emotional upsets of her partner. She often used humor appropriately to de-escalate her partner's feelings of contempt, defensiveness, and belligerence.

13 Active listening is incompatible with arguing

While active listening is outstanding during advisor–client conversations, it is actually unnatural for couples to engage in active listening in the middle of a conflict. There are times to do this, but not as a means to resolve conflicts. Asking this of couples is like requiring emotional gymnastics.

14 Gentleness and reframing

Trying to re-frame a partner's words or actions so that they are not seen as devastating allows greater amicability. For example, a client might re-frame the upset as a result of their partner's fear or some childhood event (e.g. "Adam has been so upset that our loan payment is overdue. It's probably because it reminds him of when he was a kid and his father's car was repossessed").

15 De-escalate negativity

A client in a happy marriage tends to accept their partner rather than demand change. Paradoxically, this acceptance often leads to the behavior change that is desired.

16 Marriage education is effective

The advisor can confidently recommend marriage education courses that may be offered at community centers, schools, places of worship, hospitals, etc., because they work. Brief, skills-based educational programs for couples increase marital satisfaction, improve communication skills, reduce negative conflict behaviors (including violence), and may prevent separation and divorce.[16]

ASSISTING PARENTS TO GET THEIR CHILDREN TO COOPERATE

The most common behavioral concerns that parents raise with advisors such as physicians are about their children's non-compliance, temper tantrums, and problems with eating and sleeping routines.[17] Clients will approach advisors with concerns that sound like this:

> "I'm extremely embarrassed because everyone sees that I can't handle my own child. My friends don't come by and see me anymore because of our son's behavior. He is so bad for babysitters that we have a tough time getting anyone to watch him anymore. I resent having to give up what little social life we have, and this is likely to make me hate him for a long while. I know I shouldn't feel that way, but I need to have some time for my friends and activities, and I can't seem to get it because of the problems we are constantly having with him."

This parental anguish was captured almost 30 years ago,[18] and is unfortunately as true today as it was then for too many families.

Clients in their roles as parents, grandparents, teachers, and childcare workers often feel shame and embarrassment when they struggle to get children to follow simple instructions (e.g. to come indoors for a meal, or get ready for bed). It can feel humiliating when a child does not cooperate in the more public domains (e.g. at family gatherings, parties, or on shopping trips). These clashes with adults are disturbing for the child as well. For children who appear to have special developmental disabilities, the advisor can refer the client to a specialist such as a developmental pediatrician, child clinical psychologist, or school psychologist for evaluation and treatment recommendations. However, there are many adults, whose children do not have special needs, who still struggle to get their cooperation with even the most straightforward tasks. For clients whose cultural, generational, and gender-based beliefs leave them open to asking for assistance, the advisor can help by providing insight and practical suggestions. They can begin by recommending that the client participates in one of the community-based parent education programs that are offered at such places as schools, hospitals, YMCAs, and faith-based organizations. Research has confirmed the effectiveness of such programs. A critical appraisal of 16 scientific studies concluded that despite the heterogeneity of the specific interventions, the populations studied, and the outcome measures, structured parent education programs positively influenced parents' perception that their children's behavior had improved. Furthermore, the objective measures of the children's behavior also showed positive change as a result of these structured parenting programs. These positive changes are maintained over time.[19] Parenting programs also have a positive impact on such aspects of maternal functioning as levels of anxiety, depression and self-esteem. Parenting programs have a significant effect on parenting attitudes and practices, on parental stress, and even on marriages.[20]

Adult caregivers who are kind, pleasant, and polite often approach parenting in the same way. They will gently give a child several opportunities to comply with verbally expressed parental expectations. Unfortunately, every time an adult gives a directive to a child and there is no compliance, the child learns to associate that adult's voice with not needing to cooperate. This is how adults unintentionally teach children to be uncooperative. Here is an example of such a sequence of parent directives and child responses, which the advisor can use to illustrate this point.

Mother: "Bart, would you come?"
Bart: (no response)

Mother:	"Bart, please come."
Bart:	"In a minute, Mom."
Mother:	"Bart, I'm warning you!"
Bart:	"Do I have to?"
Mother:	"Hey . . . Do what I say!"
Bart:	(finally complies)

When an adult duplicates this sequence again and again, the child learns that this individual is a "four-command" person. The client's voice unfortunately becomes a cue not to comply until four commands are given. This is independent of the gender of the parent, because it is the adult who spends the most time with the child who is the most vulnerable. In the U.S., this is often the mother. The client who is caught up in this cycle of giving reasonable directives that are not obeyed experiences a range of negative emotions, such as feeling helpless, incompetent, depressed, shamed, mean-spirited, or out of control. The adult–child relationship deteriorates. The client may love this child but find it increasingly difficult to like them, and as a result may search for ways to spend less and less time with the child. This worsens the problem. The child's non-compliant behavior may be generalized to other adults (e.g. teachers at school), and it may set up more long-term patterns. The most effective intervention for reducing non-cooperative and non-compliant behavior is to implement a new behavioral management procedure.[21]

The advisor should explain to the client that they need to use language that is clear about what is expected. It begins with an understanding that a command is not a request. A command, in this approach, is a non-negotiable item. It is something that the adult, acting responsibly, has decided must be done by the child. "No" in this case is not an option.

A request by definition means that the child has the option of saying "No." With a request, a person says "Would you . . .?" or "Please . . .", and so on. For an adult who is talking to another adult, the situation is different. An adult may say to their partner "Would you . . .?" or "Please . . ." and the other adult knows by the voice inflection and context that this actually should be done. This is not the case with children. The wise client does not assume that the child will pick up on such cues. Certainly the client can still make requests of children. They just need to accept that it is all right for the child to say "No."

Most adults just do not have the energy and time to ensure compliance with all of the commands that they typically give to their children in a day. The advisor can remind the client that for most of the time the child is not paying attention to these commands anyway. So the client should reduce the overall number of commands that they give. They should be more selective about which battles to fight. The client needs to move from four commands or so per event to one command per event. Their energy needs to be saved for making these single commands work. The wise client begins to give commands only for the most critical issues. The advisor can ask the client "What is something particularly special to you, something of sentimental value, an item so special that you would not willingly lend it for a long period of time? Would it be a particular family photograph? Would it be a piece of jewelry?" The advisor can suggest that the client should consider perceiving a command in a similar way, and regard the command as if it were as precious as that object. It should not be given away lightly.

The advisor should suggest that when the client has decided to give a command, they should walk over to the child, crouch down, and make eye contact. This means that the client can no longer call out a command from another room or yell from the inside of the home to the outside where the child may be playing. Making eye contact means that the client is committed enough to this command to leave what they are doing, walk to where the child is, crouch down in front of him or her, in direct shoulder-to-shoulder alignment, and make eye contact. If the child avoids looking at the client, the client should avoid twisting and turning to make true eye contact. When a child avoids eye contact, this means that the client indeed has the attention of the child. On no account should they tell the child to "Look at me", because that would just be to needlessly give away another precious command.

After crouching down in front of the child, and if necessary between the child and the television, the client should state the desired behavior in a simple, brief way, with a momentary pause between phrases (e.g. "Bart . . . come inside . . . now"). There should be only one command, and the client should avoid double or triple commands (e.g. "Bart . . . come inside . . . now, wash your hands . . . and start your homework"). The advisor should suggest that the client also avoids using words like "please", as that sounds like a request. There will be many occasions when the client can teach those polite words, but when giving a command is not the time. The child is not doing the client a favor by complying.

The client's tone of voice should be firm and business-like. By using this approach of reducing the number of commands, and making the commands that are given actually count, the client is less likely to become impatient, and their voice is less likely to have a loud, angry, or screaming tone.

After the command has been stated, the client should avoid a threatening staring experience. They should get up from the crouching position and count to ten silently while quietly and purposely pottering about in the area (e.g. arranging some books on a nearby shelf). This gives the child a few moments in which to "save face." It is important for the adult to ignore the child's questions about the reasons for the command. Answering such questions tends to unfairly raise false hope that the child can negotiate. It has already been determined that this is a non-negotiable situation.

If necessary, the client should ensure compliance by escorting the child to the desired location or activity. One study used such a physical guidance procedure with three 6- to 8-year-old boys who also had psychiatric diagnoses, and found that it increased compliance for all of them.[22] While escorting the child, the client should initiate some engaging and distracting banter or chatter (e.g. "You know Bart, when we're done eating I think we'll have a chance to read that story you've been talking about . . ."). Exercising good judgment should guide the avoidance of the escorting if it invokes physical aggression in older, larger children.[23] The advisor should remind the client to avoid repeating the command (e.g. by saying "I told you that you had to come inside!"), as this is just giving away that precious object again. Clients who adopt this approach to giving commands develop peace in the family because there are fewer commands given, and there is greater clarity about what are important tasks. The client him- or herself will be modeling more calm behavior.

REGAINING POSITIVE EXPECTATIONS ABOUT CHILDREN

Clients who go through long time periods when the children they care for are behaving in a non-compliant or disagreeable way can develop a negative, unhelpful bias about the children (e.g. "Mark is just so spoiled . . . he doesn't care about anyone but himself"). Pessimism about the child's ability to change may set in. Research on the concept of self-fulfilling prophecy has examined the extent to which a person's expectations about other people contributes to them performing at levels consistent with those expectations.[24] In a study of children's potential for alcohol use, perceivers' favorable beliefs had a beneficial effect on children who were at risk for negative outcomes.[25] The advisor can encourage parents, day care providers, and teachers to discipline themselves to hold realistic but favorable beliefs about the children.[26] Clients need to avoid typecasting children (e.g. "Oh you know how Anthony is, he always . . ."), because a hardening of the attitude can develop. This minimizes the likelihood of clients seeing the possibility of change ever happening. It boxes the child and client in. And it is often the point when parents will seek advice.

Clients can get out of this box and regain hope for the children. The advisor should recommend an approach in which a parent and child set aside special time to spend together.[27] One way of doing this is to use the Play-by-Play method. Here the client devotes 10 minutes each day to just be present one-on-one with the child. During this time, the client avoids instructing or guiding the child. The child chooses an activity to do in the presence of the client. The activity must be a safe one, it is the child's choice, and the client's role during this 10-minute activity is just to be with the child and to offer a supportive out-loud narrative about what the child is doing (e.g. "Oh, now you are coloring a picture of our home and the park"). The client should not advise, educate, or train the child during this Play-by-Play experience. Clients who begin to use this method regularly discover those positive aspects of the child that they have forgotten or overlooked. For example, they might start to think "I forgot how funny/artistic/curious/patient, etc. Anthony can really be." Positive expectations will re-emerge as the client realizes that the child shows more promise than they previously thought. They see the child as having engaging attributes, and they remember the child whom they used to know. As negative bias melts away, the client develops more positive expectations of the child and thus the self-fulfilling prophecy works in a positive way. This creates a much more harmonious family environment for all.

Effectively using role modeling, punishment, and praise

There are three primary approaches that clients use to influence children's behavior, namely modeling, punishment, and positive reinforcement. Modeling is one of the most powerful agents for change. It is a sobering and awesome responsibility to realize that adults raising children are never off duty. Children do as they see others do, and this includes imitating the adults in their lives. This is a part of the hidden curriculum of parenting. Children are all quietly observing how the adults in their lives manage anger, relate to alcohol and food, attend to work responsibilities, and relate to neighbors. Clients can influence children's behavior by purposefully thinking out loud about how they are handling situations. For example, a parent who is driving and is cut off by a speeding car can routinely model anger management by saying out loud "That kind of driving is just not right. It's upsetting. But I'm not going to let that cause me to lose my cool. I have to focus."

Punishment, a very popular approach, could be expressed as simply as a parent stating "Jack, because you acted in that way you lose your computer privileges for a week." The advisor should make two important points. First, punishment is best regarded as a way of getting attention. Its main effect is that it startles the child and gets their attention, but it has little actual effect on creating lasting behavioral change. A good example of how punishment can be used well is found in the sport of ice hockey. When a player has broken the rules, the official sends them to the penalty box, but only for a few minutes. The official gets the player back on the ice within a reasonably quick time, where the real behavior change happens. A player who is performing well and observing the rules gets rewarded with maximum ice time and hopefully winning plays. This same approach to punishment should be used with children. When punishment is assigned for too long a time, the learning opportunity is lost because the child forgets why they are being punished. In addition, the client is indirectly punished because they are now stuck like a prison warden monitoring the punishment. In the example given earlier, the parent must spend an entire week closely monitoring Jack to make sure that he is not sneaking in computer time, as well as having to deal with Jack's pleas for mercy. The parent also loses the option of no computer time for some other offense during that same week. Frankly, Jack's parents could get more out of suspending his computer privileges for a day rather than a week. With a briefer time period for his punishment, Jack would be more likely to remember why he was being punished in the first place. The key is to get Jack "back on the ice" as quickly as possible, so that he can have access to a procedure that really changes his behavior, and that is positive reinforcement, such as systematic complimenting.

Positive reinforcement and systematic complimenting refer to catching someone behaving well. In the culture of the classroom, large business, or the military, the leader is often responsible for managing a large group. To keep order and prevent chaos, the focus needs to be on the blips of bad behavior that appear on the radar screen. This clearly has the benefit of keeping aberrantly behaving people in line. Authority figures more rarely provide what really changes behavior, namely positive reinforcement. Paying attention to a well-behaved child is often forgotten once the child is back on the ice. When children start behaving well, they are often taken for granted. Effective positive reinforcement does not have to be an extravagant gift, such as a new computer game, in order to be effective. Systematic complimenting capitalizes on the human inclination to want to be noticed and receive attention. Clients should use it to help children to grow in a positive direction.

The following are the key points that the advisor should share with clients. The client should leave what they are doing, make eye contact with the child, and offer a few words of praise. Some clients believe that they have it covered by saying "That's terrific", "Great job!", or "Fantastic!", but fail to mention the specific behavior. Without mentioning the specific target behavior out loud to the child, that great teaching effort may be lost. The client should say those praise words and make certain that they mention the specific behavior (e.g. "That's terrific, Jack, that you came in on time!"). The client should remember that this is about encouragement, and not wait until the full desired behavior is completed before offering a compliment. They should praise the spark of change or a small positive action. If they have told the child to put their toys on the shelf, the client should begin complimenting the child when the youngster starts to move in that direction. Unlike the business-like tone of voice that is used in commands, the tone of voice for a compliment should be warm and enthusiastic. Importantly, the client should be warned against using back-handed compliments, such as "That's terrific that you came in on time, Jack. Now why can't you do that all the time?" Unfortunately, this additional piece of education, given at this time, just deflates all of the encouraging air out of the compliment balloon. The client should avoid seizing failure out of the jaws of victory.

RAISING THE 10- TO 14-YEAR-OLD: EARLY ADOLESCENCE

While there is an abundance of information about parenting babies, toddlers, elementary-school-aged children, and even youngsters of high-school age, there is surprisingly little practical information available for advising clients who are concerned about 10- to 14-year-olds, who are described as early adolescents.[28] Advisors who understand the developmental changes of both early adolescents and parents can help adult clients to have reasonable expectations of themselves and their children, still set limits, and find greater peace for their families.

The physical changes of early adolescence are easily noticed, and are often identified as the major developmental event in this age group. However, there is also an enormous growth in abstract thinking that is rarely discussed. Yet this intellectual growth is just as powerful a thunderbolt of change as the onset of physical maturity.

The thinking skills of children under the age of 10 years, regardless of how smart they are, are tied to immediate reality, to the concrete here and now. In early adolescence, these children are awakened to a new capacity to think abstractly. This new and as yet untested ability allows the early adolescent to think beyond the limits of their personal experience, and to imagine concepts such as fairness, justice, friendship, democracy, and love. This new ability to understand ideals such as equality positions them to question their parents' and teachers' views and values. Because of this growth in ability to think abstractly, early adolescents are more likely to challenge and engage in adult-type arguing. This is a significant observation that the advisor can share with a confused parent who is wondering what is the source of all these challenges.

The early adolescent now not only thinks about the football or computer game maneuver that a friend made, but also about what that friend is thinking. In fact, the early adolescent spends much time imagining what others may be thinking. Young adolescents erroneously assume that everyone else must be thinking a lot about other people, too, and especially about them. This contributes to them imagining themselves to be the center of others' attention, constantly surrounded by an imaginary audience[29] that scrutinizes their actions and appearance. Every facial blemish feels like it cannot go unnoticed. It cultivates self-consciousness, and a sensitivity to the imagined judgment of others.[30]

Feeling so conspicuous and on stage gives rise to other emotions, such as feeling uncomfortable, pressured, and even isolated. Early adolescents protect themselves from all of those eyes and ears by trying to blend in with others, and accordingly they often move around in groups. Many clients who are parents worry that their young teenager has become too self-conscious and self-centered. In truth, however, this self-absorption is a normal and natural reaction to the emergence of abstract thinking.

The young teenager's capacity to think abstractly and to engage in reflections such as "How will I fit in?" can give rise to the feeling "I must be unique or special." This common feeling during early adolescence has been termed the personal fable,[31] which refers to the stories that adolescents invent about themselves. It is characterized by over-separating one's experiences and feelings from those of others. The young adolescent is prone to believing that they are the only person who could possibly feel these intense emotions of excitement, confusion, humor, anxiety, or loss. These stories emphasize their individuality, worth, and, not infrequently, their loneliness (e.g. "I just saw the postings of who made the school baseball team, and I didn't make it. I am so ashamed. No one understands how I feel" or "I can't talk to anyone").

The personal fable may also contribute to feelings of invulnerability and risk-taking behaviors by the adolescent, who may hold the belief that "Other people might die if they tried something like this, but I'll be OK." The benefit of the personal fable is also its ability to comfort adolescents during times of stress and conflict. It can reinforce the idea that the adolescent has special value as a human being.

By the time early adolescents reach the age of 15 years, they start to accumulate reality checks and learn that they are not as much the center of others' attention as they once thought. They also begin to realize that they in fact have many feelings in common with other people, and that they are indeed vulnerable to harm as well.

Body image and physical development

The physical growth that begins in early adolescence is more rapid than growth at any other time since infancy. It is helpful for the advisor to reflect again on the basic physical changes that occur in early adolescence. For girls in the U.S., puberty begins between the ages of 8 and 13 years with the development of breast buds and the appearance of pubic hair. Menarche typically follows 2 to 2½ years after the appearance of breast buds. The mean age in the U.S. for the onset of menarche is 13 years. (Sexual development then continues with the additional development of the breasts, enlargement of the ovaries, uterus, labia, and clitoris, and thickening of the vaginal mucosa.) There is also a rapid increase in height. On average, girls reach their maximum growth velocity at around 12 years of age, approximately 2 years before boys.[32] For the first year or two after the onset of menstrual periods, the ovaries may not release an egg each month, resulting in irregular menstrual periods. The period itself evolves as well, and the amount of blood and consistency can vary. The regular adult cycle of menstrual periods may not be established until 2 years after the first period.

On average, in boys the visible signs of maturation appear later than in girls. Most boys believe that pubic hair is the first sign of puberty. However, in fact the first sign is the enlargement of the testes, usually beginning at around 12 years of age. This is followed by the appearance of pubic hair and the growth of the penis.[33] Some boys may be concerned because they feel that the absence of pubic hair means that they have not begun to develop, when in fact they are well on their way. Other important changes include facial hair growth and deepened vocal pitch, which tend to occur after the most rapid growth in height.

As a result of sexual maturation, teenagers experience many skin changes. The face and scalp become oilier, requiring more frequent bathing and shampooing. Increasing body odor, which is a result of sweat glands developing at this time, also causes concern about body cleanliness and appearance. Despite their most diligent efforts, some young teenagers may find acne and body odor difficult if not impossible to control. Not surprisingly, many adolescents have difficulty adjusting to the changes that occur within their bodies.

For both boys and girls, the rapid physical growth that occurs following the beginning of puberty can give rise to a feeling of awkwardness. This is because their growth tends to take place distally in the hands and feet before moving on to the arms, legs, and finally the trunk. This linear growth can outpace increased muscle mass, which also contributes to the experience of awkwardness.[34] Often, once young adolescents have adjusted to their new size and shape, it changes again. This challenges their efforts to maintain a stable sense of self. Their intense awareness of others their age makes them very sensitive to minor variations in their own development. Hearing from someone like a parent or healthcare provider that they are in fact quite normal and developing appropriately is very important to young people at this stage of life.

The advisor should be aware that there is much going on in the psychology of the parent as the early adolescent experiences changes. As the young adolescent grows stronger and taller, the parents may be concerned that they themselves are perhaps less strong and less tall than in their youth. When an adolescent becomes bigger and stronger than the parent, the parent may unfortunately expect more mature behavior from the youngster, and perhaps a psychological maturity that is not quite up to the level of the emerging physical stature. The adolescent is acquiring the ability to conceive children (i.e. menstruation or ejaculation), while their mother is anticipating the end of her reproductive years and the father may be concerned about his own sexual performance. Parents are also concerned about their children's sexual values, sex education, sexually transmitted infections, and adolescent pregnancy.

The world is expanding for the adolescent, and possibilities, ideas, and dreams are fascinating. Time seems like an endless resource for them. For their parents there is more of a concern about the rapid passage of time. In fact, time is measured in terms of how much longer one will live. Parents have thoughts about their legacy, concern for the continuity of their values, and a need to feel that they have contributed to the future. The adolescent's new ability to think abstractly can actually improve family communication. However, there may be tension because the child is questioning the parent's authority and testing the parent's values. The differences in time perspective between adolescents and their parents may also cause conflict.

There are different perspectives within the family that can contribute to misunderstandings. While adolescents may be losing some of their self-confidence, feeling inferior to others, and being more self-conscious and sensitive to criticism, others perceive them as moving into the highly regarded age of young adulthood. At the same time, parents may also be losing some self-confidence, and feeling inferior to others, as well as being less in control of their child, and moving into what others see as a less highly regarded stage, namely old age. Within the family there may be dynamics such as jealousy, rivalry, or mutual criticism, representing a possible conflict between inferiority complexes. While the adolescent begins to consider exciting educational, training and work roles and career possibilities, their parents are looking back on their own employment history, possibly feeling dissatisfied with their work choices and achievements. Watching their child approach decisions that have life-long implications, parents can feel responsible for giving the adolescent guidance, and concerned about his or her future employability. It is not uncommon for some parents to subconsciously want to relive their own youth through their children.

The adolescent and the parent are both attending to psychological matters outside of the immediate family. Young adolescents are looking for privacy and a degree of independence, and are concerned with what their friends think.

They become attached to friends and to adults other than their parents. Parents can be drawn to responsibilities outside the immediate family, and are adjusting to emotional losses such as the death or disability of parents or friends, as well as the empty nest syndrome. The parent–adolescent relationship moves from greater to lesser control, with the parent gradually giving (within limits) more independence. The parent or adolescent may feel conflict between letting go too early and hovering or hanging on too long. Many parents experience a sense of freedom as the adolescent becomes less dependent. The adolescent can now accept more responsibility in the family, and can begin to feel like an adult member of the family. The parents can develop a new identity that incorporates their physical, intellectual, and social changes. There may be a shift in the roles of husband and wife as new options open to the parents. For example, one parent may increase their out-of-home work responsibility, or the parent who is least involved with the adolescent may actually become more involved through some recently identified shared interests. Other changes may also occur during the adolescent stage, such as a parental death or divorce.

In conclusion, the advisor should remember that puberty hits a child like a hormonal thunderbolt. And lightning does strike twice, with the second thunderbolt being a powerful growth in abstract reasoning. With this new tool, these young people now think about what others are thinking, and they make the error of believing that others are often thinking about them. This gives rise to feelings of conspicuousness, and the need to reduce this by conforming with peers. The growth in abstract thinking also allows these young people to access such feelings as justice and fairness, and they consequently offer challenging arguments to their parents. Simultaneously, the parents are experiencing their own developmental growth by recognizing a gradual changing of the guard, trying to graciously protect their children while gradually letting go, and accepting with wisdom their new roles as the emerging elders in the family and community.

REFERENCES

Helping troubled marriages and relationships

1 Burman B, Margolin G. Analysis of the association between marital relationships and health problems: an interactional perspective. *Psychological Bulletin* 1992; **112**: 39–63.

2 Dawson D. *Family Structure and Children's Health: United States, 1988. Series 10: Data from the National Health Survey No. 178.* Washington, DC: Centers for Disease Control, National Center for Health Statistics, US Department of Health and Human Services; 1991.

3 Harknett K. *Children's Elevated Risk of Asthma in Unmarried Families: underlying structural and behavioral mechanisms.* http://crcw.princeton.edu/publications/publications.asp (accessed 1 March 2008).

4 Troxel W, Mathews K. What are the costs of marital conflict and dissolution to children's physical health? *Clinical Child and Family Psychology Review* 2004; **7**: 29–57.

5 Umberson D, Williams K. Marital quality, health and aging: gender equity? *Journals of Gerontology, Series B: Psychological Sciences and Social Sciences* 2005; **60**: 109–13.

6 Coyne J, Rohrbaugh M, Shoham V *et al*. Prognostic importance of marital quality for survival of congestive heart failure. *American Journal of Cardiology* 2001; **88**: 526–9.

7 Gallo L, Troxel W, Kuller L *et al*. Marital status, marital quality, and atherosclerotic burden in postmenopausal women. *Psychosomatic Medicine* 2003; **65**: 952–62.

8 Kielcolt-Glaser J, Newton T. Marriage and health: his and hers. *Psychological Bulletin* 2001; **127**: 472–503.

9 Staton J. *What is the Relationship of Marriage to Physical Health?* Fairfax, VA: National Healthy Marriage Resource Center; 2008.

10 US Bureau of the Census. *Statistical Abstract of the United States, 2002 (122nd Edn)*. Washington, DC: US Government Printing Office; 2006.

11 Ibid.

12 Ganong L, Coleman M. *Stepfamily Relationships: development, dynamics, and interventions*. New York: Kluwer Academic/Plenum Publishers; 2004.

13 Grizzard T. Love in the time of medical school. *American Family Physician* 2002; **66**: 907–8.

14 Gottman J, Coan J, Carrere S *et al*. Predicting marital happiness and stability from newlywed interactions. *Journal of Marriage and the Family* 1998; **60**: 5–22.

15 Gottman J. *The Marriage Clinic: a scientifically based marital therapy*. New York: WW Norton & Company; 1999.

16 Stanley S. Premarital education, marital quality, and marital stability: findings from a large, random household survey. *Journal of Family Psychology* 2006; **20**: 117–26.

Assisting parents to get their children to cooperate

17 Albrecht S, Dore D, Nagle A. Common behavioral dilemmas of the school-aged child. *Pediatric Clinics of North America* 2003; **50**: 841–57.

18 Barkley R. *Hyperactive Children: a handbook for diagnosis and treatment*. New York: Guilford Press; 1981.

19 Barlow J, Stewart-Brown S. Behavior problems and group-based parent education programs. *Developmental and Behavioral Pediatrics* 2000; **21**: 356–70.

20 Barlow J, Coren E, Stewart-Brown S. Parent-training programmes for improving maternal psychosocial health. *Cochrane Database of Systematic Reviews* 2001; **Issue 2**: CD002020. DOI: 10.1002/14651858.CD002020.pub2.

21 Wilder D, Atwell J. Evaluation of a guided compliance procedure to reduce noncompliance among preschool children. *Behavioral Interventions* 2006; **21**: 265–72.

22 Tarbox R, Wallace M, Penrod B *et al*. Effects of three-step prompting on compliance with caregiver requests. *Journal of Applied Behavior Analysis* 2007; **40**: 703–6.

23 Wilder D, Atwell J, op. cit.

Regaining positive expectations about children

24 Jussim L, Harber K. Teacher expectations and self-fulfilling prophecies: knowns and unknowns, resolved and unresolved controversies. *Personality and Social Psychology Review* 2005; **9**: 131–55.

25 Willard J, Madon S, Guyll M *et al.* Self-efficacy as a moderator of negative and positive self-fulfilling prophecy effects: mothers' beliefs and children's alcohol use. *European Journal of Social Psychology* 2008; **38**: 499–520.

26 Eden D. OD and self-fulfilling prophecy: boosting productivity by raising expectations. *Journal of Applied Behavioral Science* 1986; **22**: 1–13.

27 Barkley R. *Defiant Children: a clinician's manual for assessment and parent training.* New York: Guilford Press; 1997.

Raising the 10- to 14-year-old: Early adolescence

28 Short M, Rosenthal S. Psychosocial development and puberty. *Annals of the New York Academy of Sciences* 2008; **1135**: 36–42.

29 Elkind D. Egocentrism in adolescence. *Child Development* 1967; **38**: 1025–34.

30 Dacey J, Kenney M. *Adolescent Development.* Madison, WI: Brown & Benchmark Publishers; 1994.

31 Elkind D, op. cit.

32 Hazen E, Schlozman S, Beresin E. Adolescent psychological development: a review. *Pediatrics in Review* 2008; **29**: 151–68.

33 Ibid.

34 Ibid.

Bad news, violence, and grieving

DELIVERING BAD NEWS

Some clients want advice on how to communicate bad news, and an advisor can help with this. Bad news has been defined as "any information which adversely and seriously affects an individual's view of his or her future."[1] This could be, for example, the death of a loved one, a serious medical diagnosis, a family member's decision to divorce, a teacher's report of a child doing very poorly at school, or a job loss. What is considered bad news is always determined by the recipient. News that may seem routine and relatively ordinary for one person may be experienced as a crushing blow by another.

Much research about how to deliver bad news humanely comes from the medical field, and these experiences help with non-medical life events as well. Eggly and colleagues[2] suggest that clients should be prepared for all interactions in which they will disclose information to a person, from the apparently most momentous to the apparently most trivial, because any news could be experienced as stressful or bad. The preparations should include confirming for oneself the facts, rehearsing if this is an unfamiliar task, and arranging for adequate time and privacy. The protocol should include eliciting the recipient's perspective, respecting the recipient's right to decide whether and what they want to be told, sharing manageable amounts of information in a paced way, and attending to the tone as well as the content of the delivery.

One approach to communicating bad news, which is called SPIKES, involves Setting up the interview, Perception of the recipient, Invitation, Knowledge, Empathy, and Strategy.[3] It can be summarized as follows.

1 Setting up the interview ahead of time

The client should invite the people whom the recipient wants to have present, ensure that the necessary information is available, arrange for privacy, and provide adequate seating and tissues. They can reduce the tension to some extent by inviting everyone to sit down (which signals a readiness to listen and talk), letting everyone know how much time is available for the discussion, and avoiding interruptions by arranging to have calls and pagers dealt with by others during that time.

2 Perception of the recipient

Because of their anxiety, some clients might rush to tell the bad news without checking what the recipient may already know. The advisor should suggest a simple opening comment such as "Tell me what you understand so far about what is going on." The recipient may say "I understand that I have lung cancer, and I'll need surgery" or "I heard that Adam may be separating from Eve." The client can then validate, clarify, or correct this information accordingly. The client may hear about a person's emotional state at this time as well (e.g. "I've been so worried about Eve that I haven't slept for a week").

3 Invitation to hear a level of detail

The client should ask how much information the recipient wants to be given at this time, because ethnicity, family tradition, culture, religion, and socioeconomic class create individual differences here. And as time progresses, this may change in different ways. The client needs to remember that each person has the right to voluntarily decline information, and may designate someone else to communicate on his or her behalf. Not everyone wants to know all the details. In medicine, for example, having a conversation at the time when medical tests are ordered can be helpful (e.g. "When the test results come back, how much would you like me to share with you?"). In the workplace the client could make a similar enquiry (e.g. "The company's economic forecast looks bleak for the coming fiscal year – what kind of information would you like to know?"). The advisor can suggest that the client uses the following kind of question: "Some people want me to cover every detail, while others prefer only the big picture. What would you prefer now?" This establishes that there is no right answer, and that it is acceptable for different people to have different preferences. The client can also mention that the door will remain wide open for additional questions later. They could say "If this turns out to be something serious, do you want to know?" or "Some people really do not want to be told what is wrong, but would rather their families be told instead. What would you prefer?"

4 Knowledge given in a paced manner

The advisor should recommend that the knowledge is imparted in a paced, sensitive manner. Before telling the bad news, the client should first provide a warning shot. The recipient needs to prepare to hear the bad news, and a warning lessens the shock. The client could make a statement such as "I wish I had better news for you." The client should then give the bad news in small sound bites, avoid bluntness and technical jargon, and check the recipient's understanding. This will minimize the likelihood of anger being directed at the client as the bearer of bad news. When the medical, economic, or social news is not good, the client can always give hope by offering to be there to provide loyal support, technical advice, and additional resources.

The client should prepare to answer questions from everyone present. In the outpatient oncology setting, for example, research has shown that those who gave bad news found that the patient's companions actually asked significantly more questions than the patient, as 38% of the questions were asked by the patient and 62% of the questions were asked by companions.[4]

5 Empathy with the emotions of everyone involved

The client should directly ask "How do you feel about what I have told you?", and then show support by making an empathic response. The advisor should explain that regardless of how humanely the presentation has been orchestrated, the recipient may express or repress a range of emotions, some of which may sound extreme, such as anger, disbelief, and despair.

6 Strategy

The client should then provide a strategy and give a verbal summary of the discussion. People who receive bad news tend to feel better when they know what the next steps will be.

Bad news can also be humanely shared by using the WATER model, which involves Warning, Awareness, Thirst, Education, and Reaction. The following is an example of the use of this approach.

➤ **Warning:** This helps the recipient to prepare for the shock of the news (e.g. "Mr. Gonzales, the report is back . . . I wish I had better news", followed by a pause).

➤ **Awareness:** This identifies the information that the recipient already knows. This helps the client to share the relevant information and relevant clarification (e.g. "Mr. Gonzales, tell me what you understand about your symptoms, and what a colonoscopy can show us").

➤ **Thirst:** This asks how much should be shared and with whom (e.g. "Some people want to know all the information, and some don't. Some people want certain family or friends to be here, too. What would you prefer, Mr. Gonzales?").

➤ **Education:** Here the client delivers information in logical and reasonable chunks, provides support, and offers hope by recommending the next steps (e.g. "Mr. Gonzales, I feel badly to have to tell you this. As you and I had discussed earlier, the growth did turn out to be cancer. In my experience, there's unfortunately no question about the test results. It's cancer." . . . pauses . . . "I will make sure you receive all the care that you need, including prescribing the right medicine to help you feel comfortable. I will be with you every step of the way. In a moment I will answer all your questions."

➤ **Reactions:** There will be emotional reactions that should be identified (e.g. "How are you feeling as you hear this?").

It is important to be cautious about a natural tendency at this point to say "I'm sorry", which may be misinterpreted as indicating that the client in this case is responsible for the situation. If the goal is to show empathy, it is best expressed as "I'm sorry to have to tell you this." The client should give the news simply and briefly, and then stop. They should avoid delivering all of the information in a single, steady monologue, and pause frequently, finally suggesting a simple next step. The advisor needs to tell the client that once the person hears the bad news, the torch has passed from the cognitive to the emotional. No matter how well crafted the client's words are, the recipient is probably not really available to absorb much more information. Even those recipients who may appear attentive are probably emotionally flooded and will not absorb more information until there is some emotional validation. The client needs to ask how the recipient is feeling. If the recipient can express feelings, then perhaps something might be heard. If it is necessary to bring closure to the expression of feelings, the client can ask a cognitive question such as "What is your main concern right now about this news?" The client should next communicate an understanding of the recipient's questions, and present a plan. With a plan there is hope. For a client who is a medical provider, that hope could be in the form of another diagnostic test if this is appropriate. Or it could be assuring the recipient that the medical team will assist with pain management. It could involve assuring the recipient that the client will be available long term to answer questions and provide follow-up care. At this point, the client would propose a plan that addresses the recipient's concerns (e.g. "Here are the ways we are going to handle things. We will have the cancer doctors see you this afternoon, Mr. Gonzales. In the meantime, we are going to aggressively help you manage the pain. And I think your thought of getting a second opinion is an excellent idea. I will be with you every step of the way"). The client should be explicit about when the next contact will be (e.g. "I'm going to ask our receptionist to call you, and I want to see you no later than Tuesday. Again, I will continue to be with you every step along the way. Is there anything else I can do for you right now, Mr. Gonzales?").

It is possible that a family member might say, for example, "Don't tell my mother what is wrong with her." While it is a physician's legal responsibility to obtain informed consent from the patient, an effective therapeutic relationship requires a congenial alliance with the family. Rather than confronting the family and saying "I have to tell the patient", the client should ask them to explain their concern, and find out what they believe will be said. The client should inquire about what the recipient's past experience has been with bad news, and ascertain whether their concern has a personal or cultural context. The client can suggest that the family member and the client go to the patient together to ask what he or she wants to know. Most often the justification for family members not wanting the patient to know what is wrong with them is commendable, as the family wants to spare the patient a painful or difficult experience. However, these fears are usually unfounded. In rare situations, the family may reveal that telling the truth will cause the patient extreme distress, or may cause predictable harm to the patient. In those situations, it may be appropriate to withhold the information. Most often, however, telling the truth in a thoughtful and empathic manner will be more appropriate than withholding information.

Is the withholding of bad news ever justified? The competent patient might ask not to be told the results or the truth. It may be important to treat this like an informed consent. The patient should be notified about the consequences of not hearing the bad news. If those consequences are accepted, the patient's wishes not to know should be honored.

What if the patient is a child, and the parents do not want the child to know? This protective instinct is understandable, but may ultimately be problematic. As the child experiences treatments and procedures, they will inevitably perceive that there is a problem. The child may feel distrustful and misled when this happens, and it could compromise care. To avoid this situation, a better initial plan may be to help the parents to understand that this is likely to occur.

These situations may require significant negotiation. In particularly difficult cases, healthcare providers can ask for input and support from the institution's ethics committee. Unless the recipient has previously indicated a preference not to be given information, concealing the diagnosis or withholding important information about the prognosis or treatment is neither ethical nor legally acceptable. Physicians do not need to feel constrained to practice in a way that compromises care or seems unethical. If the physician and the patient's family are not able to agree, the physician may choose to withdraw from the case and transfer the care of the patient to another physician.

Delivering bad news includes but goes well beyond medical concerns. The following is an example of how a client, Suzanne, used the WATER approach to share with her husband Mark the bad news that she had lost her job.

Warning:

Suzanne:	"Mark, the annual fiscal report was announced at work today. I met with Mr. Quinn, the big boss . . . (pause) . . . I wish I had better news."

Awareness:

Suzanne:	"Mark, you look upset, what have you heard?"
Mark:	"I heard that some people are being laid off and that there is no severance."

Thirst:

Suzanne:	"How much of what Mr. Quinn told me do you want to know?"
Mark:	"I want to help you, tell me everything."

Education:

Suzanne:	"Mark, I feel so bad having to tell you this. Just like we thought, I got laid off. I know the timing, with Robin going off to college, is really bad. But I have some ideas about how we can handle this."
Mark:	"I'm sorry, Suzanne. I want you to know we will be OK. I'll just get another job if I need to. And you'll be back on your feet soon. You're just too good at what you do."

Reactions:

Suzanne:	"I know I feel awful. How are you feeling about all this?"
Mark:	"I'm worried."
Suzanne:	"What is your main concern right now about this news?" . . . (pause)
Mark:	"Like you, I'm worried about having enough to pay for Robin's tuition."
Suzanne:	"Here are some ways I think we can handle things . . . Mr. Quinn did say that I'd get severance for 3 months, and that he'd help me get a position with our other office."

VIOLENCE AGAINST WOMEN

Some clients who are being abused will trust an advisor enough to tell their story. It is confusing and bewildering for the client, and can also confuse and bewilder the advisor. A knowledge of the spectrum and prevalence of violence against women, the characteristics of women at particular risk, how the cycle of violence inhibits some women from leaving, and skills that encourage clients to disclose violence, are all competencies that steady the advisor. Although nearly all physicians believe that the identification and management of family violence is important, in actual practice asking about this serious problem is uncommon. Most physicians believe that abuse is not common in their practice. They believe that asking about violence will damage their relationship with the patient, that they have insufficient training, and that they have too little time to ask questions about violence in any case.[5]

So while healthcare providers are encouraged to ask about violence, other advisors need to fill the ranks and ask women clients about this. Language is important here, because in much of the literature the term being used is "abuse" or "domestic violence." This usage is a problem because when violence is described as "domestic", women's experience disappears behind that of all those for whom they care, including children, adolescents, siblings, the elderly, and the disabled. It is important for the advisor to distinguish violence against women from other forms of family violence, such as child and elder abuse. Battered women's needs are different from those of battered children and battered elderly people. It is important for the advisor to accept the fact that most battered adults are women, and most batterers are men."[6]

Violence against women is a common problem. Women who are single, pregnant, poor, teenagers, or young adults, and who have a history of abusing alcohol and drugs, are at particular risk. The advisor should be vigilant when a woman client talks about a partner who seems to be excessively jealous or possessive, or even when a restraining order exists, because not all men who abuse women honor such directives. One in four women seeking care in an Emergency Department for any reason is a victim of domestic violence, one in six pregnant women are abused during pregnancy, one in four women have been abused at some point in their life, one in seven women report having been abused within the preceding 12 months, and one in four women who are treated for psychiatric symptoms have been battered.[7]

In one survey of the prevalence among patients in a family practice setting,[8] 11% of the women who were currently in important relationships had been hit or hurt by a partner in the past year, and 35% had been hit or hurt during their lifetime. Among the men who were currently in important relationships, 7%

reported having hit or hurt their partner in the past year, and 16% had hit or hurt someone during their lifetime. Among those men and women who were currently in relationships, 26% of the men and 42% of the women reported current or lifetime physical violence in their relationships, which involved either hurting their partners or being hurt, or both.

Advisors' and clients' understanding of what constitutes abuse is unfortunately often limited. Abuse is most commonly only identified if physically assaultive behaviors are present, such as slapping, punching, kicking, pinching, biting, grabbing, choking, restraining, pulling the hair of the victim, and sexual assault. Clients' confusion about what they are experiencing can be clarified when the advisor explains that there are other behaviors that are also abusive. These include the perpetrator destroying furniture and possessions, and injuring pets. Abusive behavior also includes controlling or coercive behavior, such as when a perpetrator withholds money, a car, or health insurance, refuses to pay bills, sabotages the woman's attempts to work or go to school, harasses the woman by making uninvited visits or phone calls, or sending her unwanted letters, text messages, and emails, and embarrassing the woman in public. Some perpetrators intimidate through implicit or direct threats or criticism of the victim. They may use weapons, throw objects, stand and block the doorway or corner the woman during arguments, shout, swear, or drive recklessly. Some perpetrators isolate the woman by restricting and tracking her activities and use of the telephone, or threaten her by stating their intent to seek custody of or kidnap the children, or they may threaten to kill the victim or themselves.

Men who abuse women come from all racial, religious and socioeconomic backgrounds. They objectify women and do not consider them worthy of respect. They see women as sexual objects or even as their property. During the courtship period, the man may rush into intimacy, convincing the woman that she is the one and that he cannot live without her. Once he has captured her, the process of exercising control over her behavior, freedom of movement, and even her thinking begins.

Advisors who help to stop abuse also eliminate the training grounds for future problems when the children are grown. This is because the witnessing of domestic violence is the single best predictor of drug abuse, juvenile delinquency and engaging in multiple health risk behaviors.[9] When boys witness violence against women, they learn that males are violent and do not respect women, and as adults they are 10 times more likely to use violence on their partners. Girls learn that male violence is normal, and tend to accept it in adult relationships. Exposure to poor modeling in the electronic entertainment industry may play a role as well.[10]

Abused women are clear about what they want from advisors such as physicians.[11] Nearly all of the women surveyed wanted their doctors to ask about family conflict and believed that physicians can be helpful. Unfortunately, only one-third of the women reported that their physician had ever asked them about family conflict. These women recommended that the advisor should gently inquire about the possibility of violence, even if the woman appears to be uninterested. The advisor should first establish a comfortable and safe relationship, and should then ask the following two questions:[12] "Do you ever feel unsafe at home?" and "Has anyone at home tried to hit you or tried to injure you in any way?" These two questions have a sensitivity of 71% and a specificity of 85% in detecting domestic violence.

Another screening approach uses the PEACE acronym:[13]

➤ Physical: Have you ever been in a relationship in which you have been Physically hurt by a partner or someone you love?

➤ Eggshells: Have you ever felt that you were walking on Eggshells to avoid conflicts with a partner or someone you love?

➤ Abuse: Have you ever been sexually Abused, threatened, or forced to have sex, or to participate in sexual practices when you did not want to?

➤ Control: Has your partner or someone you love tried to Control where you go, what you do, who you talk to, or who your friends are?

➤ Emotional: Have you ever been Emotionally abused or threatened by a partner or someone you love?

If any of these screens are positive, the client should encourage the woman to talk about the issue, and should listen without judging her. This begins the healing process for the woman, and yields information that serves as a guide to how to help her further. The advisor should be assertive but must avoid being pushy, demanding, or patronising towards these women, who are probably experiencing some shame. Many advisors find it easy to initially empathize with a woman who is being abused. The challenge is to maintain that empathy when the advisor's suggestions seem to go unheeded and the woman chooses to stay with her abusive partner. Some inexperienced advisors start out well meaning, but can become insistent and judgmental. Unfortunately, this can actually mimic the dynamic of the abusive relationship. The women who were surveyed[14] also made it clear that the advisor needs to be ready to listen, and to provide emotional support and information about local resources. The advisor should keep in mind that regardless of the exact words or language that they use, it is more likely that genuine empathy and respect will carry the day. So the advisor should empathize, validate, and offer hope (e.g. "You are not alone", "You don't deserve to be treated this way", "You are not to blame", "You are not crazy", "What happened to you is a crime", "Help is available for you").

The advisor can help to maintain empathy by appreciating that if the woman could easily and safely remove herself from such a situation, she would do so. There are reasons why women feel that they have no other option but to stay in an abusive relationship. Some women may see abuse as a common feature of family life, having grown up in a home where it was natural for a father to beat those he loved, such as his wife or children. Financial dependence is a major reason for staying within an abusive relationship, as some women may not be able to work because of childcare responsibilities, a lack of transportation, or a lack of marketable skills. For some, government assistance is meagre or non-existent, and they need the abusive man's financial support. If the woman was to report the abuse, her partner might lose his job, which would mean that there would be no income to support her and possibly her children. Therefore some women make a personal pact to remain victimized in order to ensure some financial security for themselves and their children.

Fear is a powerful weapon for the perpetrator, who may cultivate an image as all-powerful, influential, resourceful, and connected, persuading the woman that there is no real way to protect herself. She may fear that his extended family or connections will take revenge on her. Isolation is common, with the abuser having systematically destroyed the woman's support system of friends, so that he is the only psychological support she has left. And she may have little idea that other support services may be available. Learned helplessness and low self-esteem set in as the woman may have tried to leave many times without success. It is very difficult to keep striving when many previous efforts have come to naught. Depression can result from this situation. Religious and cultural beliefs relate to violence against women as well. Women may have ingrained beliefs about what they see as their duty and responsibility in an adult relationship. This may include personal, societal, and extended familial pressures to maintain the façade of a good marriage, such as staying for the sake of the children.

The advisor can help to reduce the woman's confusion and restore some of her sense of control by explaining the features of a common, repeating cycle of abuse.[15] Each phase is characterized by relatively predictable behaviors for the abuser, the woman, and her experience of denial. The phases are as follows:

➤ tension building
➤ acute explosion
➤ honeymoon period
➤ re-cycle back to the tension building.

During the tension-building phase the abuser is moody, nitpicking, critical, sullen, and threatening, begins to withdraw affection, starts to isolate the woman, begins to drink or take drugs, and destroys property. The woman responds by trying to agree with him, to calm him, and staying away from her family and friends. She tries to keep the peace by being nurturing towards him, cooking his favorite dinner, keeping the children quiet, and walking on eggshells. Her denial manifests itself by her blaming the situation on an outside force such as herself, his job, traffic, or his drinking.

This phase is followed by an acute explosion in which the abuser engages in such behaviors as hitting, choking, humiliation, imprisoning, rape, verbal abuse, using weapons, beating, and blaming the situation on the woman (e.g. "She had it coming"). The woman responds by protecting herself in any way that she can, by calling neighbors and the police, leaving, and continuing to try to calm the abuser.

She engages in denial by such behaviors as saying that her injuries are only minor (e.g. "I bruise easily"). She continues to avoid blaming the abuser. Instead, she again assigns blame to other influences (e.g. "He was upset because he was laid off from work" or "He was having a few beers with his friends and didn't really mean it"). She does not describe sexual assault as rape because it was her husband.

This is followed by the honeymoon phase. The abuser starts to say "I'm sorry", declares his love for her, cries, begs forgiveness, sends her flowers, brings her presents, enlists family support, wants to make love, or promises to go to counseling sessions or to religious services. He may even believe that the abuse will not happen again. The woman responds by agreeing to stay, to return home, or to take him back. She starts to feel happy and hopeful again, she stops legal proceedings, and she may start setting up counseling appointments for him. Her denial continues to manifest itself as she minimizes her injuries (e.g. "It could have been worse"), believes the abuser's promises, and believes that this particular period of safety and peace will be permanent ("He really is a good man deep down"). Then the tension-building phase begins once again, soon to be followed by the acute explosion, and so the vicious cycle continues.

For women with physical injuries, the advisor should recommend a thorough physical exam,[16] which should include a urogenital examination that would show evidence of forcible rape or violent insertion of foreign objects. If the patient is pregnant, the healthcare provider can look for signs of abdominal trauma and rule out possible injury to the fetus or uterus. The next step of course is to treat the injuries. The physician or healthcare provider should document these injuries particularly carefully. If the medical record and testimony are in conflict in court, the medical record may be considered a more reliable source. Healthcare providers can use the format "The patient states . . ." Details of the injuries, such as size, number, pattern, and possible cause, are important. The healthcare provider can also use a body map and, with the client's permission, a photograph of the injuries can be taken before medical treatment is given. If the client's explanation is inconsistent with the nature of the injury, the documented observations will be particularly important. For example, a woman may state that she fell down the stairs, but her injuries include a pattern of bruises on her neck, and might be noted in the record as "possible intentional injury." The healthcare provider should indicate whether the police have been called, and include the name(s) of the responding officer(s).

The healthcare provider should assess the level of danger to the woman, such as an increase in the frequency or severity of the assaults, increasing or new threats of homicide or suicide by the abuser, threats to her children, and the presence or availability of a firearm. The healthcare provider should also provide appropriate treatment, referral, and support, and of course treat the patient's injuries as indicated. When prescribing medication, the healthcare provider should keep in mind that certain medications may hinder the woman's ability to protect herself or flee. It is important that the advisor and the healthcare provider ask about the availability of safe refuge, and that they understand that it may be dangerous for the woman if she has written information in her possession.

As suggested earlier, women survivors of abuse need advisors to actively participate in lifting the veil of shame and secrecy from their abuse. Advisors can give them hope that they can gain control and create a life that is free from abuse. This requires a team effort. An advisor can help by supportively listening to the survivor's story, educating them about the cycle of violence, alerting them to local agencies that deal with violence against women, and helping to connect them to healthcare providers who can treat their injuries compassionately.[17] If possible, the advisor should close these conversations by offering a follow-up meeting.

IDENTIFYING YOUNG PEOPLE AT RISK FOR VIOLENCE

This section will close with a brief discussion of youth violence, which is another major concern in many schools, neighborhoods, families, and workplaces. Clients may seek advice in order to help to identify a young person at risk for violent behavior. Advisors can help by knowing the risk factors that place young people in harm's way for engaging in violence. The following approach is based on the acronym MD STAT. The client should be alert for Moodiness. This can include moving from anger to sadness to happiness, as well as a feeling of despair, a lack of positive expectations, a feeling of being persecuted, and a tendency to act impulsively. The client should also determine whether the young person is involved in Drugs and Defiance. This includes alcohol use as well as the use of illicit drugs. The defiance includes a pattern of not listening to authority as well as behaving in a significantly oppositional way at school and elsewhere. Self-absorption is another warning sign, and is characterized by a young person who hardly seems to speak to others, has few friends, and ignores the feelings of others. Truancy from school (or academic failure) is another sign, as is Attraction to violence, such as having been involved in a fight in the last 12 months, being obsessed with weapons, death, or violence, and writing about these subjects. Threatening others in person, on the phone, or electronically is of particular concern, especially if the threats include specific plans. Positive observations on Drug use, Truancy (or academic failure), Attraction to violence, and having been involved in a fight in the last 12 months are particularly correlated with subsequent violence-related injury.[18]

Again, family violence appears to be self-perpetuating. A child who grows up witnessing violence against others in the family or who is a victim of violence is particularly at risk for developing a tendency towards violent behavior. A sociological perspective has yielded the following model[19] of how a child grows up to become violent. The child is first physically abused or brutalized. They then have no other option but to be a victim or to strike back. The youngster who does strike back violently, and who is successful in this, gains respect and is in fact coached to develop this skill. The growing child then makes a decision to use violence from that time onward. This parallels the spirit of W.H. Auden's[20] poem:

> I and the public know
> What all schoolchildren learn,
> Those to whom evil is done
> Do evil in return.

HEALTHY GRIEVING

Clients who are grieving a loss, such as the death of a loved one, will approach an advisor for guidance, reassurance, and comfort. The advisor who is alert to the markers of healthy, normal grieving and unhealthy, prolonged grieving will be well equipped to help. A classic study by Zerbe and Steinberg[21] forms the basis of many of the following recommendations. There is a biopsychosocial reaction to any loss, including but not limited to a loss of a life, physical health, a job, a home, a relationship (through divorce), and so on. Common features of these reactions are separation distress (e.g. feeling sad and angry), traumatic distress (e.g. feeling absolute disbelief), survivor guilt (e.g. feeling remorseful), and social withdrawal.

Bereavement is the internal grief that is specific to the loss of a loved one. It has been described as the price that is paid for loving someone. Mourning is different. It is the external behavioral and social manifestation of bereavement. It includes the work that is associated with grief. This involves the cultural and religious rituals and activities, such as methods of dealing with the clothes of the deceased and settling their finances. Depression can get in the way of doing this work. Treating depression, if it is present, helps people to recover from both the depression and the grief.

Acute grief is painful and preoccupying, but it is also temporary. And it is clearly the most common reaction. However, because research on chronic grief has historically dominated the literature, it has given the erroneous impression that prolonged acute painful reactions are the norm.[22] In fact, some and possibly many bereaved clients will exhibit little or no grief, and these clients are not cold, unfeeling, or lacking in attachment. Rather, these are clients who are capable of genuine resilience in the face of loss.[23] Research studies have shown that such individuals score highly on pre-bereavement measures suggestive of the ability to adapt well to loss, such as an acceptance of death or a belief in a just world. The majority of these resilient individuals certainly experience some yearning and emotional pangs, intrusive thoughts and ruminations at some point early after the loss. However, these feelings are transient and do not interfere with functioning in other areas of their lives, including their capacity for positive emotion.[24] The informed advisor can reassure the many clients who handle death fairly well that this is a normal reaction. They can encourage them not to feel guilty if they do not feel miserable. Research on the adjustment of widows and widowers[25] has established the best current understanding of normal bereavement. In this study, 350 men and women in their early sixties were interviewed at home within 2 months of the death of a spouse. About 14% of the participants had a history of major depression, and in 63% of the cases, death was expected. They were then followed up by questionnaires that were administered at 6, 12, 18, and 24 months.

A yearning for the deceased spouse was a common emotional response of the surviving partner.[26] This feeling was common initially, but it decreased in intensity and frequency over time. Although popular culture might lead clients to expect a step-wise staging of grief (e.g. denial, anger, bargaining, depression, and acceptance[27]), the process of grief does not necessarily unfold in this theoretically predicted way. Instead, all of those feelings are present initially, but they then lessen in intensity and frequency over time. In fact, positive emotions and behaviors are also common, including talking about the deceased spouse, recollections, telling amusing anecdotes, taking pride in honoring the deceased, warmth in recollecting the closeness of the relationship, and relief from the burden of caring for the deceased. Some clients will feel guilty about having positive feelings, and will find that talking about this with the advisor will relieve the guilt. Clients who experience more positive feelings immediately after the loss tend to do better over time. Positive emotions also relate to pre-loss resilience and post-loss life satisfaction, tranquillity, and optimism.

Maintaining a relationship with the deceased spouse is a common and fundamental part of healthy grieving. Rather than death severing the attachment, the successfully grieving client maintains and reformulates the attachment and keeps the deceased person in their life both psychologically and emotionally over time. For example, approximately 66% of survivors felt that the deceased spouse was watching over them in some way, and approximately 50% felt the same way after 2 years. At 2 months, 39% of survivors were talking regularly to the deceased spouse, and 23% were still doing so after 2 years. The frequency of dreaming about the deceased spouse actually increased over time, as the survivor found ways to accept the loss during their waking hours. Symbolic representation, such as keeping the belongings of the deceased, was reported by 48% of survivors at 2 months and 36% at 2 years. Hearing the voice of the deceased is not pathologic hallucination, but is a natural part of maintaining the relationship.[28]

Advisors need to know what is normal or healthy about starting new relationships, as survivors and family members will raise this question. Immediately after the loss, most men felt that they would never be attracted to another woman. This feeling changes with time, as 61% of the men who were studied were in a new relationship or actually remarried by 2 years.[29] The factors that predicted which men would develop a new relationship or remarry included having financial resources and higher education. Women were less likely to develop new intimate relationships or to remarry, because they were less interested, they were more loyal to the deceased spouse, and there was simply a shortage of men in older age groups. The only predictor for developing new relationships or remarrying was young age of the woman. If depression was present, both widows and widowers were less likely to develop a new relationship or to remarry. Advisors should encourage the family members and friends of the widowed to be respectful, supportive, and encouraging, as widows and widowers who enter into new relationships fare better and tend to be less depressed, and these new relationships tend to be successful.

Research indicates that people who have lost a loved one experience an increase in general medical morbidity after that loss, and individuals with a history of drug or alcohol abuse are at higher risk of a recurrence or exacerbation.[30] No widows or widowers started using drugs or alcohol if they had not used them before. In fact the functioning of widows and widowers usually improves over time, and it is important that the advisor reassures the client about this. People often report that having been married, having dealt with grief and having survived makes them feel stronger, more sensitive to others, and more self-confident. In fact, 2 months after the loss, 62% of people who have lost a loved one feel that they are adjusting well, by the first anniversary of the death that figure reaches 70%, and by 2 years after the death it is 75%. The following model of a normal bio-behavioral process, which can be helpful for organizing the advisor's thinking, has emerged from this research.[31]

Immediately after the death of a loved one there is an acute grief reaction. After approximately 6 months the acute grief reaction lessens, as survivors experience some degree of acceptance, feel more positive emotion, forgive themselves, develop compassion, and begin to attribute meaning to the loss. The acute grief reaction is replaced by an integrated grief or abiding grief. The loss has now moved from the foreground to the background of the person's awareness. The background state can be prompted to re-emerge into a foreground state by anniversaries, reminiscences, or happy occasions that the survivor would have liked to have shared with the deceased.

In addition to reassuring the client about the likely normalcy of their grieving process, the advisor can show support in the following ways. Taking the initiative is important. Rather than saying "Call me when you need to talk", the advisor should state "I'll call you tomorrow afternoon." The advisor should listen, express sympathy, encourage the client to express their feelings, acknowledge that they cannot know exactly what the person is going through, inquire about the circumstances of the death, talk about the deceased and mention the deceased by name, and send a condolence card (because such cards can be very comforting). The advisor should ask the bereaved person's permission to attend the funeral or memorial service, and if that is acceptable they should certainly attend. The advisor should avoid saying that the death was for the best or somehow acceptable, or that the bereaved person is strong and that they will or should get over it.

Although transition from an acute grief reaction to an integrated grief is the most common experience, there are some clients who experience a prolonged acute grief, which is also known as unresolved, complicated, or traumatic grief. This prolonged acute grief is considered to present when the acute grief symptoms persist at 6 months. This kind of chronic depression and distress may occur in 10–15% of bereaved individuals.[32] Instead of accepting the death, attributing meaning to their loss, and developing new relationships, these individuals have a predominant emotional experience of fear. They fear psychological pain, loss of control, being considered disloyal, and losing their self-identity. A disbelief about the death persists. Anger and guilt are excessive and directed at almost anyone, including the client him- or herself, the deceased person, God, caregivers, and the doctor. The client with prolonged acute grief feels indignation, engages in rumination and excessive avoidance, and just does not progress on to the healthy state of integrated grief. If the client does not get some help for this, prolonged acute grief can last for years. It is a painful and disabling condition that hinders both the development of new relationships and the maintenance of existing relationships. Prolonged acute grief is also associated with poor health and multiple other comorbidities, including an increased suicide risk. One of the ways to manage prolonged acute grief is through a psychotherapeutic approach known as combined grief therapy. In these sessions, the client works hard both on coping with the grief and pain and on restoring a satisfying life. This is addressed by setting personal goals, working on interpersonal problems, and revisiting satisfying activities and places. Research has shown that those clients who were taking antidepressant medicine had better adherence rates for the combined grief therapy, and had the best outcomes.

Acute grief is painful and disruptive, but usually evolves into a less painful, integrated grief. Acute grief is not a medical condition. The majority of people who have lost a loved one progress through grief well and do not require treatment. Advisors can provide significant emotional support by demonstrating sympathy and empathy as well as normalizing the survivor's expectations. The advisor should be alert to identifying complications such as prolonged acute grief, and in such cases should help the client to get appropriate treatment by referring them on for psychotherapy and medication evaluation.

REFERENCES
Delivering bad news

1 Buckman R. *How to Break Bad News: a guide for health care professionals*. Baltimore, MD: Johns Hopkins University Press; 1992.
2 Eggly S, Penner L, Albrecht T et al. Discussing bad news in the outpatient oncology clinic: rethinking current communication guidelines. *Journal of Clinical Oncology* 2001; 24: 716–19.
3 Baile W, Buckman R, Lenzi R et al. SPIKES – a six-step protocol for delivering bad news: application to the patient with cancer. *Oncologist* 2000; 5: 302–11.
4 Eggly S, Penner L, Albrecht T, op. cit.

Violence against women

5 Burge S, Schneider F, Ivy L *et al.* Patients' advice to physicians about intervening in family conflict. *Annals of Family Medicine* 2005; **3**: 248–53.

6 Flitcraft A. Clinical violence intervention: lessons from battered women. *Journal of Health Care for the Poor and Underserved* 1995; **6**: 187–97.

7 Eisenstat S, Bancroft L. Domestic violence. *New England Journal of Medicine* 1999; **341**: 886–92.

8 Burge S, Schneider F, Ivy L *et al.*, op. cit.

9 DuRant R, Smith J, Kreiter S *et al.* The relationship between early age of onset of initial substance use and engaging in multiple health risk behaviors among young adolescents. *Archives of Pediatrics and Adolescent Medicine* 1999; **153**: 286–91.

10 Pelcovitz D. Psychiatric disorders in adolescents exposed to domestic violence and physical abuse. *American Journal of Orthopsychiatry* 2000; **70**: 360–69.

11 Burge S, Schneider F, Ivy L *et al.*, op. cit.

12 Feldhaus K, Koziol-McLain J, Amsbury H *et al.* Accuracy of 3 brief screening questions for detecting partner violence in the emergency department. *Journal of the American Medical Association* 1997; **277**: 1357–61.

13 Kirk H, Weisbrod J, Ericson K. *Psychosocial Aspects of Medicine.* Philadelphia, PA: Lippincott Williams & Wilkins; 2002.

14 Burge S, Schneider F, Ivy L *et al.*, op. cit.

15 Walker L. *The Battered Woman Syndrome.* New York: Springer; 1984.

16 Kirk H, Weisbrod J, Ericson K, op. cit.

17 Ibid.

Identifying young people at risk for violence

18 Sege R, Stringham P, Short S *et al.* Ten years after: examination of adolescent screening questions that predict future violence-related injury. *Journal of Adolescent Health* 1999; **24**: 395–402.

19 Rhodes R. *Why They Kill: the discoveries of a maverick criminologist.* New York: Alfred A. Knopf; 1999.

20 Auden WH. September 1, 1939. In: *Another Time.* 1st edn. New York: Random House; 1940.

Healthy grieving

21 Zerbe K, Steinberg D. Coming to terms with grief and loss: can skills for dealing with bereavement be learned? *Postgraduate Medicine* 2000; **108**: 97–106.

22 Bonanno G. Loss, trauma, and human resilience: have we underestimated the human capacity to thrive after extremely aversive events? *American Psychologist* 2004; **59**: 20–28.

23 Bonanno G, Wortman C, Lehman D *et al.* Resilience to loss and chronic grief: a prospective study from pre-loss to 18 months post-loss. *Journal of Personality and Social Psychology* 2002; **83**: 1150–64.

24 Ibid.

25 Zisook S, Shuchter S. Uncomplicated bereavement. *Journal of Clinical Psychiatry* 1993; **54:** 365–72.

26 Ibid.

27 Kubler-Ross E. *On Death and Dying.* New York: Macmillan; 1969.

28 Zisook S, Shuchter S, op. cit.

29 Ibid.

30 Ibid.

31 Ibid.

32 Bonanno G, Wortman C, Lehman D *et al.,* op. cit.

Thriving at work

DEVELOPING LEADERSHIP SKILLS

Moving onto greater responsibilities at work, in the family, or in the community is gratifying and exciting. Some clients will feel overwhelmed by their new responsibilities, realizing that they must master new competencies, ration their time, triage and prioritize new demands, and further develop effective supervisory and leadership abilities. These clients can feel adrift, self-doubt can emerge, and because they want confidentiality, they may only share these concerns with an advisor. The advisor can help the client to feel better organized by using the metaphor of the captain of a sailing ship. By considering and understanding the roles of a successful captain,[1] using the acronym CAPTAIN as described below, the client can become better organized to guide and lead the crew on a successful and productive voyage.

The successful captain has **Concern** for the crew and their safety as their number one responsibility. The successful captain plans a voyage of reasonable time length and difficulty so that the crew's efforts can be successful. The captain ensures crew members' safety by being vigilant. He or she anticipates weather changes and makes adjustments if necessary, keeps an eye out for boats that can help as well as harm, and looks for sharks.

The successful captain **Assigns** key roles to the crew members. This enables the work to get done, and it also cultivates shared leadership, fosters loyalty, and builds morale. The successful captain then empowers the crew members by getting out of their way so that they can learn to problem solve on their own and thus grow in competence and confidence.

The successful captain **Provides** the right material, equipment, tools, and provisions so that the crew members can be safe and successful.

The successful captain **Trains** new members of the crew by direct instruction in the appropriate knowledge, attitude, and skills. They also train the crew by being an intentional role model for the way things should be done, they give positive and negative feedback, and they ask questions to allow the crew to practice quick thinking. The successful captain accomplishes this by adopting a manner that is encouraging and ego-empowering, and avoids shaming the crew.

The successful captain is **Adventuresome**. This may have its origin in a leader's dissatisfaction with the status quo or doing things the same old way. The successful captain makes the voyage fun and exciting for all. There is a search for some chop in the waves and exciting and unique places to explore.

The successful captain is **Inspirational**. Such captains have ways of effectively sharing an exciting vision of what is possible. Crew members work hard for a captain who gives them hope that together they will be able to achieve great things. The crew also benefits from their growing conviction that this particular captain's leadership will help them all to get there.

The successful captain **Notices** the activities of the crew at first hand, rather than hearing about what is happening through another source. And they observe the crew doing well and can then offer specific, positive, and enthusiastic feedback.

TAILORING THE SUPERVISION

Advisors can share the fact that successful leaders tailor their supervisory and instructional style to meet learners' individual developmental needs. A style of supervision that works with an inexperienced employee needs to be changed to fit the needs of a more veteran worker. The same holds for parents as they raise their children, who are also changing ages and stages. Some parents are skilled in teaching their young children, but struggle with how to teach the children as they grow more competent. Some adults in the workplace find themselves skilled at supervising experienced employees, but less skilled at handling those who are new to the job.

Clients will ask for help with their supervisory roles. The advisor should suggest that the client should first establish the learner's stage of competency and level of interest in learning. The following model of competency, popularized by Gordon Training International, emerges from such concepts as the Johari Window.[2] A knowledge of this *awareness of skills model* will help the client to adjust their teaching style accordingly. There are four developmental stages, with each stage signaling the use of a different teaching approach matching the learner's developmental needs. Learners may be:

1 *Unaware of their lack of skills.*
   This is particularly challenging because the learners do not know what they

do not know. Because they are naive and probably clueless about their deficits, there is little incentive for them to change. Here the supervisor has to give feedback about these deficits that will lead to the next stage.

2 *Aware of their lack of skills.*
After the supervisor has informed the learners that their work needs improvement, the learners become somewhat anxious. This is a healthy and appropriate level of performance anxiety, because it motivates learners who want to succeed. These learners now realize that they have to achieve more in order to succeed. There is a shift in their motivation. They are now highly committed but have a low level of competence. A learner might be thinking "This is the first time I have ever worked in such a job and place. I'm really motivated and psyched up to do well, but I don't even know where the bathroom is!"

At this stage, the supervisor's responsibility is to direct the learner. This means providing specific instructions and closely supervising the task being done (e.g. "Take this package down this hall to the executive suite. It's on the left in Room 23. And give it to Kate, she's the vice-president").

3 *Aware of their good skills.*
Learners at this stage are performing well but a little awkwardly. They have to consciously focus on sequential, concrete steps. They need to operate in a deliberate, step-by-step fashion in order to do well. The learner has now acquired some skills, and will therefore be less anxious and perhaps even a bit less motivated (e.g. "I've been able to find Kate and get these reports to her on time, even when she is not in Room 23. I understand my role. I'm far ahead of where I was back in July. I hope my supervisor respects that").

At this stage, the supervisor should adopt more of a coaching style. They continue to direct and closely supervise the learner, but now also explain their decisions, ask for suggestions, and support the learner's progress (e.g. "When Kate is not in the building to receive these packages, you can deliver them to Jack. I need your input – are there any other ways in which we can improve our efficiency?"). The supervisor respects the fact that the learner is growing in competency and can contribute helpful suggestions (e.g. "I think it would work best if on Tuesdays I just deliver the packages to Jack, because I know Kate is scheduled for a meeting then at the main office").

At this stage of the learner's development, the supervisor facilitates the learner's problem-solving skills and begins to share responsibility for decision making. The supervisor reinforces the learner's progress and asks for the learner's opinion (e.g. "You've really been efficient with distributing our materials. Do you think we should get Nora, Lorenzo, and Jackson involved?").

4 *Unaware of their good skills.*

Here learners have so over-learned the skill that they have reached an automatic, smooth, and almost effortless level of performance. The learner is highly competent. They are also highly committed to deepen their competencies and develop more skills because they realize that soon autonomous and independent functioning will be expected (e.g. at this stage they might think "I've distributed all the packages. Everything is in order. Soon I'll be on my own with all this. I'd better ask all my questions while I still can").

The supervisor who recognizes this stage will prepare the learner by delegating and turning over decision-making responsibilities (e.g. "I know distribution operations are in good hands with you being in charge. I'm going to Brooklyn Heights, Princeton, Chicago, and then to San Francisco to visit our most important customers. I know you can handle things. You can always reach me if you want my opinion").

GIVING FEEDBACK EFFECTIVELY

As clients move up the ranks at work, their responsibilities for observing supervisees' activities and giving them feedback will likely grow. Clients will ask the advisor for help because the process of giving feedback can be challenging, uncomfortable, and create significant anxiety. One reason for this is that supervisors are rarely taught ways to provide feedback effectively.[3,4] For example, learners often receive brief and non-specific feedback, such as "I agree" or "Right."[5] Supervisors also tend to overestimate how effectively they give feedback. One study showed that although 90% of supervising/teaching surgeons reported that they were giving feedback successfully, only 17% of their learners agreed with that claim.[6] Supervisors and learners can feel a range of negative emotions, such as feeling unenthusiastic or anxious, as they anticipate giving or receiving feedback. For this reason many people avoid asking for or giving feedback. Learners then lose opportunities to find out how they can improve, and the entire crew loses out. Contrary to the belief of many supervisors, the evidence suggests that learners still desire and value feedback.[7]

The advisor can learn concepts and techniques that can help clients. In fact, some of these clients, as part of their assigning role, may even have to teach others how to effectively provide feedback. Clients who are supervisors can learn to provide both positive and negative feedback in a spirit of unconditional positive regard, and in a way that is clearly designed to help to improve the learner's performance.[8]

The advisor should explain that feedback is about a mutually shared understanding between two people, namely the learner who wants to advance in knowledge, attitude, or skill, and the supervisor who agrees to help the learner to get there (e.g. to learn to use the computer system efficiently). In a sense it is indeed a training or education agreement. Learners, like Olympic-level speed skaters, are appropriately fully immersed in their work. Understandably, they are unable to view their performance from various distances and angles. Like a good speed-skating coach, the leader has a wider view from different angles, and can share that information. This information is a gift. The learner can receive it and use it to get to the desired goal.

The advisor should make it clear that feedback is not the same as evaluation. This is often an upsetting cause of confusion. The confusion regarding an agreed-upon definition of feedback also makes scholarship in this area challenging.[9] Feedback is really just information about what was done. It is not the annual evaluation or performance review for considering a salary increase. That is quite different. Evaluation assumes that a reasonable amount of time has elapsed since the feedback was given, so that the learner has had a chance to make performance changes to be successful by the time of the agreed evaluation date. With evaluations, most often there is a formal written report that is completed by some fixed date (e.g. the last day of the fiscal year, or the date of the learner's annual salary review). Learners react differently to feedback from the way they react to evaluation. This is because evaluation implies a mandatory response. The learner must conform because the loss of a job or a promotion may be at stake. Evaluation brings with it the image of an academic grade, or a comparison, or a judgment.

Unlike evaluation, feedback is non-judgmental.[10] As described in one of the classic articles on feedback,[11] good feedback is an informed, non-evaluative, objective observation of a person's performance. Feedback implies a choice on the part of the recipient. Because feedback is non-judgmental, both the supervisor and the learner are on a relatively equal footing in the communication. The learner is not obligated to change their behavior in the way that they would have to do as a result of an evaluation.

Positive feedback is information that helps learners to see what they are doing that is bringing them closer to their goal. Negative feedback helps learners to see what they are doing that is taking them further away from their goal. It is useful if at the beginning of a complex work or learning task, the leader and the learner agree that both positive and negative feedback will be helpful, and to expect this as a way to achieve the goal. Feedback helps learners to adjust their performance as necessary to be successful before the actual evaluation takes place.

The advisor can share effective ways of giving feedback. Feedback is best offered when the performance is fresh (e.g. at the time when the activity is taking place or soon afterwards). It should be limited to one or two items, to avoid overwhelming the learner,[12] and it should be limited to only those items over which the learner has control. Feedback should also be restricted to what was directly observed. The supervisor should avoid using judgmental language[13] or tone of voice. The anticipation of providing feedback brings up such uncomfortable images and feelings because many clients have received feedback that, in terms of language and voice tone, was disrespectful, exaggerated, and embarrassing. Receiving feedback that is delivered in a demeaning way is annoying, and can lead to some occupational self-destructiveness. The learner may act passive-aggressively, retrench, and avoid improving just out of spite. The advisor can teach the client the Describe, React, and Predict procedure as a professional and respectful way to provide an appropriate level of feedback.

The Describe level is a reminder that for many situations, all that is needed is to describe what was observed and share this without interpretation or evaluation. This protects the supervisor from unnecessary, lengthy, and uncomfortable mini-lectures that could be misinterpreted as attacks on the learner. The learner often just gets it at this point and can take it from there. If that level of feedback is not effective, the supervisor can go to the next level and add React by expressing an emotion. If the React level does not seem to penetrate, the supervisor can go to the next level and add Predict, which concerns what might happen if the change does not take place. The following is an example of how this procedure works.

➤ **Describe** what was observed: "I noticed that you arrived at 9.30."
➤ **React** with an emotion: "I noticed that you arrived at 9.30 . . . and I am concerned."
➤ **Predict** what might happen if the behavior continues: "I noticed that you arrived at 9.30 . . . and I am concerned . . . if this continues, the director could suspend you."

All three levels of feedback are appropriate, and it just depends upon what the supervisor feels is needed at the time. When the learner is not absorbing the less invasive observations, the supervisor can step it up to the next level of feedback to get the learner's attention. The wisdom and good judgment of the supervisor are important, because the supervisor needs to decide how invasive to be. All of this rests upon the assumption that the relationship between the supervisor and the learner is an educationally healthy one, with the learner wanting feedback in order to progress. Another important competency is including the Describe,

React, and Predict procedure in a more complete, educationally supportive conversation, such as that discussed below.

The language of feedback should be practical, clear, free from evaluative words and provided in a private, relaxed and supportive climate. It should end with an offer to meet again for follow-up.

The supervisor should start the feedback conversation by asking for the learner's own observation. Not only will this communicate respect, but the learner's own observation often captures the information that the leader wanted to share anyway. The supervisor simply asks "How do you think it went?"

Next, the supervisor asks the learner to share specific, positive details by asking "What do you think went particularly well?" The supervisor then inquires about the learner's ideas about negative specifics, by asking "What do you want to improve upon?" The supervisor then summarizes the learner's own self-feedback.

Now is the time for the supervisor to offer some feedback. The skilled supervisor asks if the learner wants to hear another observation (e.g. "Can I tell you what I've observed?" or "Shall I give you some feedback? I think it will help you"). They then offer feedback, using one of the Describe, React, and Predict levels. The supervisor closes by checking to what extent the feedback was clear and understood.

The process of giving feedback may be the most important skill that clients can use in their leadership roles at work. The advisor who can share how to do this effectively can greatly reduce many clients' anxieties and apprehensions in the workplace. These skills also help in respectively communicating with family members and friends. It is through feedback that people can see whether they are making progress towards the goal that they want.

SPEAKING UP EFFECTIVELY IN GROUPS

A survey of randomly selected residents in a medium-sized Canadian city investigated which of a series of proposed social situations made people feel most anxious.[14] The number one fear was public speaking. This fear did not diminish when the proposed size of the crowd was reduced or even when the proposed level of ease with the participants was increased, since speaking to a small group of familiar people came in second in the rankings. Clearly too many people feel incompetent and under-confident about making such presentations. This affects clients' careers. However, advisors can offer suggestions that will help to lower this fear and anxiety.

Successful speakers recognize that it is less about what they want to discuss and more about what the target audience wants to learn. Whether it is the client's supervisors, co-workers, guests, or members of a community or religious group, to be more competent and thereby confident, the client needs to determine what is meaningful and important to this group. They should then craft a goal that matches the group's interest. This should be ambitious and inspiring. For example, the goal of a presentation could be "to develop speakers who will motivate adolescents to lead psychologically healthy lives." Once the client has articulated a meaningful goal for the presentation, the advisor should explain the importance of crafting objectives that are clear and measurable.[15] While the goal is deliberately passionate and grand, objectives obligate the client to state the ways in which the audience should have been altered by the end of the speech. If the audience has not changed in some specific ways, learning has not taken place, and the whole exercise has been pointless. Forming objectives helps to prevent this from happening. Successful speakers commit themselves to measurable objectives to change the participants' knowledge, attitudes, or skills. A knowledge objective uses verbs such as "list", "discuss", "describe", or "compare." An attitude objective uses verbs such as "commit", "advocate", "defend", or "persuade." A skill objective uses verbs such as "assemble", "implement", "perform", or "deliver." Having too many objectives for a presentation can cause the client to lose focus in both the preparation and delivery. It can confuse the audience and trigger daydreaming. Vollman[16] has written about the importance of limiting a presentation to no more than five key messages, and most often three actual objectives are sufficient. Well-crafted objectives also include a target number. Having target numbers protects the client from being over- or under-ambitious, and helps them to stay within the prescribed amount of time set aside for the presentation. Including a target number within each objective also allows for a pre- and post-talk comparison if a formal evaluation of the presentation is desirable. Here is an example.

> At the end of this presentation, the participants will be able to:
> 1 (Knowledge) Name at least three tips to improve PowerPoint slides
> 2 (Attitude) Commit to using at least one relaxing technique before making a speech
> 3 (Skill) Write at least one clear objective for a speech.

For present purposes, this example used an objective from each of the knowledge, attitude, and skill domains. Based upon what works best with their goal, the client will decide whether they want a change in two attitude domains and one knowledge domain, or three knowledge domains, and so on. Once the objectives have been defined, the advisor should recommend that the client uses self-discipline to adhere to these three or fewer objectives during the preparation of the content and pedagogical style of the talk (e.g. showing a movie clip, audience involvement, etc.). Establishing objectives is a very effective time management tool, as it minimizes the client's tendency to go off on a tangent. This reduces their preparation anxiety. Outstanding speakers adjust the objectives as the presentation is being prepared, because they often realize that the time allocated for the component parts may permit only two of the objectives to be presented. Or the client might realize that what originally looked like one objective is in fact three combined into one, and it needs to be broken down.

When the goal and objectives have been clearly defined, the advisor should recommend the next step of determining how to shape the remarks and visuals so that the objectives can be met in the time allocated. If a slide or PowerPoint presentation is planned, the speaker should be careful about visual density. Each slide should be planned as a billboard, not a bulletin board.[17] In other words, the PowerPoint slide should attract attention rather than supply all the details. So for each slide the client should use the 5-7-7 rule – no more than five words in the title, seven words in a line, and seven lines of text.[18] Because audience members visually tend to track from their left to their right, the client should be positioned on the left side of their visual field, and the PowerPoint or visual aid should be on their right. The client should avoid reciting what is on the slides. If the slide is that important, the client may be regarded as irrelevant. Instead, they should speak from the notes with spontaneity, and at times with passion, adding personal observations, sharing stories, answering participants' questions, and occasionally breaking up the visuals with some pictures.

In terms of actual oral presentation skills, the client speaker should maintain eye contact with the participants, as this is the most important quality upon which a presentation is judged. Using a strategy for eye contact is one of the best secrets to relaxing oneself as a speaker and connecting with members of a small committee as well as a large audience. One way to achieve this self-relaxing effect is to hold a person's gaze while completing a full thought, and only then to move on to make eye contact with another person and complete a full thought with that person. It gives the effect of a real conversation going on between the speaker and the full audience. Making eye contact in this manner helps the speaker to maintain a conversational tone. With a large group, the client should begin by looking at a person at the back of the room, then make eye contact with a person at the front, and then a person at the extreme left and right, as these people in particular are often excluded from a speaker's attention. The best way to be energized, spontaneous, and passionate is to practice. The aim is for the client to avoid repeating what is on the slide verbatim, because the audience can read for themselves. The presence of the client should add something quite different to aid the learning. The client should know the material and teaching method well enough to flexibly interact with the audience. It has been recommended that it may take up to 10 hours of preparation for each hour of presentation.[19]

Before speaking, the client can also reduce tension by letting go of a deep breath. They can then relax their shoulders slightly, smile, and while standing allow their arms to hang at their side. If this is a more formal presentation, the person can begin with a "social handshake", by welcoming and/or thanking the audience for coming, and genuinely acknowledging the expertise of the audience in a collegial way. As part of the social handshake the speaker can provide personal context by briefly introducing him- or herself in a friendly manner. Using stories, anecdotes, and case examples allows the audience to connect with the speaker. As appropriate, the speaker can get the audience to laugh.

Finally, if possible the speaker should end each lecture at or before the allocated time. This will be an unexpected gift for the audience, and they will be eternally grateful.

HANDLING COMPLAINTS AND CRITICISMS

At work as well as at home, it is difficult for people to be on the receiving end of complaints and criticisms. Too often a client who is receiving legitimate complaints and criticisms becomes immediately defensive, causing the other person to feel dismissed and to react by heightening the vitriol, possibly repeating the criticism, trying to fight through what is perceived as denial. Clients can learn to maintain a respectful relationship with their supervisor and thereby be able to share a perspective in a manner that might actually be heard. In a marriage or a work situation, not being able to react coolly under the pressure of a complaint or criticism can cause more serious problems. This is an important topic for advisors, because some clients will avoid work or home because they do not know how to comfortably respond to such criticisms. When there is good faith and some legitimacy behind the complaint or criticism, the advisor can recommend the See, Sorry, and Say method. This can be summarized as follows:

➤ "I can **See** what you are talking about."
➤ "I'm **Sorry** you are so upset."
➤ "If I can **Say** what I think happened it might help . . ."

This method asks the client to resist the temptation to contest the other person so quickly. Rather, the client acknowledges the other person's position. The critic or complainer, depending on their mood state, can then feel validated. Only then does the client have an opportunity to express a point of view that could be heard.

➤ **See:** "I see what you mean, Lauren, not calling the office right away caused us to miss setting up that appointment."
➤ **Sorry:** "I'm sorry about that."
➤ **Say:** "I was trying not to bother Sheila and David so early in the day. Sounds like I don't have to be concerned about that."

One of the most difficult experiences to handle is when a customer or even a co-worker makes hurtful or inappropriately critical remarks. Clients can become clinically depressed or anxious when they are regularly exposed to chronically disagreeable and mean-spirited co-workers or customers who criticize them and put them down. Many clients avoid saying anything, concerned that they would impulsively blurt out something inappropriate to defend themselves, and that there would be a retaliatory action. Yet such behavior by a family member or co-worker can be intimidating and possibly abusive. Some clients feel repressed. They over-think what to say, how to say it, and over-plan for the best time to say it, without accomplishing anything. This approach becomes the unhelpful "Ready, Ready, Ready, Aim, Aim, Aim, and possibly Fire" approach. These clients never get round to responding to the criticism. Or when they do respond, the actual incident is by then history. The advisor can call a person's attention to this and recommend the "Fire, Aim, Ready" approach. Such situations may need to be handled quickly and with a no-nonsense verbal response (e.g. "That's enough, Frank" or "That's not how I see it, Frank"). If the remark is a mean-spirited complaint or vicious comment, the person can simply say "We're done, Frank."

When clients practice this with the advisor and start doing it for real, they learn that they can survive being assertive, and often the other person begins to back down. If such efforts do not cause a change in the client's attitude or the other person's behavior, the client may have to decide whether this other person has a pathological problem that merits other kinds of solutions, such as getting help for depression and/or leaving this toxic work or family environment long term for a newer and healthier environment.

REFERENCES
Developing leadership skills

1 Clabby J. Winslow Homer's 'Breezing Up': inspiring providers of community primary care. *Family Medicine* 2004; **36**: 321–3.

Tailoring the supervision

2 Luft J, Ingham H. *The Johari Window: a graphic model for interpersonal relations.* Los Angeles, CA: University of California Western Training Laboratory, UCLA; 1955.

Giving feedback effectively

3 Salerno S, O'Malley P, Pangaro L *et al*. Faculty development seminars based on the one-minute preceptor improve feedback in the ambulatory setting. *Journal of General Internal Medicine* 2002; **17**: 779–87.

4 Quirk M, Stone S, Chuman A *et al*. Using differences between perceptions of importance and competence to identify teaching needs of primary care preceptors. *Teaching and Learning in Medicine* 2002; **14**: 157–63.

5 Jackson J, O'Malley P, Salerno S *et al*. The teacher and learner interactive assessment system (TeLIAS): a new tool to assess teaching behaviors in the ambulatory setting. *Teaching and Learning in Medicine* 2002; **14**: 249–56.

6 Sender-Liberman A, Liberman M, Steinart Y *et al*. Surgery residents and attending surgeons have different perspectives of feedback. *Medical Teacher* 2005; **27**: 470–72.

7 Dobbie A, Tysinger J. Evidence-based strategies that help office-based teachers give effective feedback. *Family Medicine* 2005; **37**: 617–19.

8 Ibid.

9 van de Ridder J, Stokking K, McGaghie W *et al*. What is feedback in clinical education? *Medical Education* 2008; **42**: 189–97.

10 Wood B. Feedback: a key feature of medical training. *Radiology* 2000; **215**: 17–19.

11 Ende J. Feedback in clinical medical education. *Journal of the American Medical Association* 1983; **250**: 777–81.

12 Cantillon P, Sargeant J. Teaching rounds: giving feedback in clinical settings. *British Medical Journal* 2008; **337**: 1961.

13 Ibid.

Speaking up effectively in groups

14 Stein M, Walker J, Forde D. Setting diagnostic thresholds for social phobia: considerations from a community survey of social anxiety. *American Journal of Psychiatry* 1994; **151**: 408–12.

15 Kelly MH. *How to Teach an Old Dog New Tricks: training techniques for the adult learner*. Des Plaines, IL: American Society of Safety Engineers; 2006.

16 Vollman K. Enhancing presentation skills for the advanced practice nurse: strategies for success. *AACN Clinical Issues* 2005; **16**: 67–7.

17 Stein K. The dos and don'ts of PowerPoint presentations. *Journal of the American Dietetic Association* 2006; **106**: 1746–8.

18 Vollman K, op. cit.

19 Hindle T. *Making Presentations*. New York: Springer; 1997.

Commencement

It takes a village to promote psychological and behavioral health. Depending on where families live, there may be mental health insiders available who are licensed or certified to provide psychotherapy or counseling services. The advisor can refer clients to licensed psychologists, family physicians, psychiatrists, licensed social workers, certified professional counselors, nurse practitioners, certified alcohol counselors, or pastoral counselors. Professionals in each of these specialties may be found in independent private practice as well as on staff at the agencies found in many communities. Yet non-professionals are often the first line of defense. Knowing how to listen well and offer specific advice is a formidable combination. As stated in the preface to this book, the world cannot afford to disenfranchise the many adults who with additional information can begin to relieve psychological and behavioral suffering with two minute talks.

Index